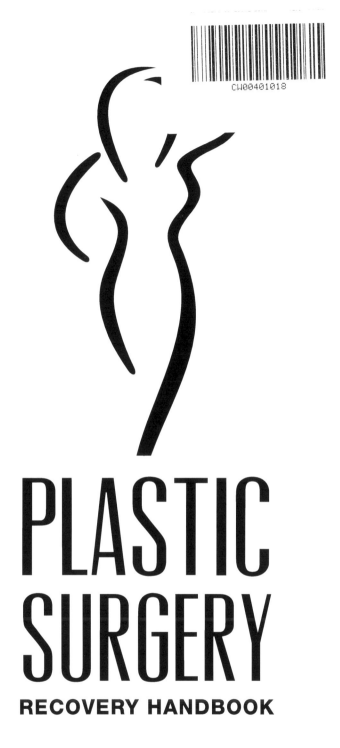

PLASTIC SURGERY

RECOVERY HANDBOOK

KATHLEEN HELEN LISSON, CLT

Disclaimer and Terms of Use

No information contained in this book should be considered as medical advice. Your reliance upon information and content obtained by you at or through this publication is solely at your own risk. Solace Massage and Mindfulness or the author assumes no liability or responsibility for damage or injury to you, other persons, or property arising from any use of any product, information, idea, or instruction contained in the content or services provided to you through this book. Reliance upon information contained in this material is solely at the reader's own risk. The author has no financial interest in and receives no compensation from manufacturers of products or websites mentioned in this book.

ISBN-13: 978-1-7328066-3-4

ISBN-10: 1-7328066-3-2

CONTENTS

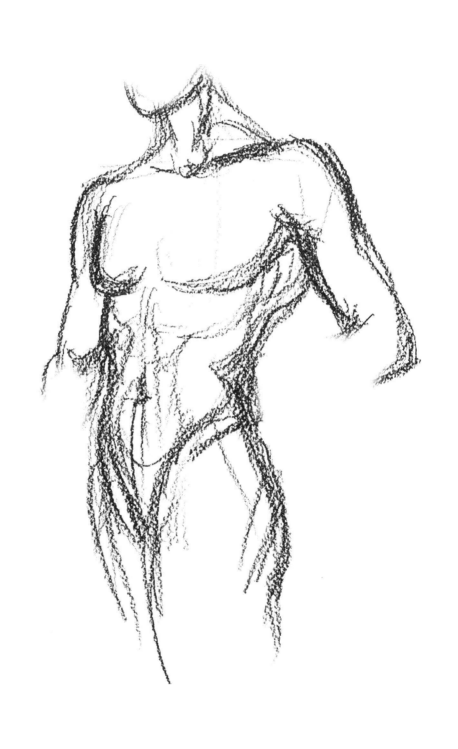

IMPORTANT NOTES

The tips discussed in this book were compiled through reviewing research studies and published literature on plastic surgery, interviewing experts, and listening to clients. Experts may disagree and scientific advances may render some of this information outdated. The author assumes no responsibility for any outcome of applying the information in this book for self-care. If you have any safety-related questions about the application of techniques discussed in this book, please consult your physician or plastic surgeon.

Quickstart Guide

CHAPTER 1
WHY I WROTE THIS BOOK

Congratulations! You have just had plastic surgery to improve your appearance.

Isn't it frustrating that before you can begin to enjoy your new face or body, you must spend days or weeks feeling swollen and bruised?

Many of my clients ask me why I limit my massage practice to just people who have swelling after surgery. How do I empathize so well with how they are feeling: scared, frustrated and maybe even a little angry at themselves or their bodies?

It's because I have followed the path you are on myself.

What have I had "done"?

I had two different types of surgery on my face, and I wish someone had told me about lymphatic massage after my operations.

The tale of my first plastic surgery started on the side of a ski slope in Western Massachusetts. I was in my thirties and had gone skiing on a warm February day. I was on a "green" hill, taking my time, and skied over to one side to let the woman behind me pass me by.

I watched her coming, coming, coming and SMASH.

She hit me on my right side, and I crumpled to the ground. I was rescued by the ski patrol, strapped onto a toboggan, hauled down the mountain, and driven by a friend to the ER in my hometown later that day. The verdict: my face was swollen and bruised, my right cheekbone was shattered, and I needed reconstructive surgery.

Thanks to **Dr. Stephane Braun**, my surgery was successful, but I was told the swelling and bruising was normal and that the best thing to do was to wait patiently for my body to heal itself.

What did you just say? You've heard that from your doctor, too? We're not alone. Doc is right: swelling is a normal part of recovery from trauma, including plastic, reconstructive, oncologic, and orthopedic surgery, but there ARE ways to reduce swelling and heal faster.

Whether it was in person or online, we connected with one another because you have swelling, too. Board Certified Plastic Surgeons in San Diego, across Southern California, and in Tijuana, Mexico, refer their clients to me to reduce the heavy, tight feeling that postoperative swelling can bring. Even if you're not my client, you can still benefit from this advice!

I will share my top tips picked up from my training as a Certified Lymphedema Therapist, conversations with fellow therapists, presentations at lymphedema conferences, books, research studies, and helpful hints shared by my clients about what has worked best for them.

First, let me introduce my seven key components to healing from plastic surgery. Based on years of experience helping clients, I believe addressing each of these components boosts the chances of healing fully from surgery.

Components of Postsurgical Recovery Therapy

- Follow Doctor's Orders
- Reduce Swelling
- Reduce Bruising
- Reduce Scars and Fibrosis
- Support Wound Healing
- Get Back on Your Feet
- Feel Healthy Inside and Out

Each of the following chapters will explain in detail how to follow my recovery rules. Let's get started!

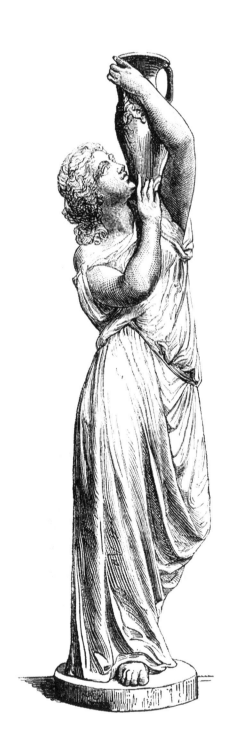

CHAPTER 2
FOLLOWING DOCTOR'S ORDERS

I created this book as a resource to jumpstart and support a conversation about your plastic surgery recovery with your surgeon.

Yes, your surgeon wants and values your input in your recovery!

In their book *Breast Augmentation and Body Contouring*, Doctors McNemar, Salzberg, and Seidel say "cosmetic surgeons consider it your responsibility as a patient to be informed, to ask questions, to communicate your goals, and to follow instructions" (2006). Most of the advice in this book is backed by research, and I have put links to most of the studies in the bibliography so you can print them and show them to your physician.

In their book *Cosmetic Surgery for Dummies*, Dr. R. Merrell Olesen and Marie B.V. Olesen share that "you can influence the healing process positively by choosing to follow your surgeon's instructions and by getting lots of rest" (2005). Let your doctor have the final say in your treatment decisions; they have knowledge of your unique case.

To ensure you are healing as quickly as possible, let's review your plastic surgeon's recommendations for your recovery. What are the answers to these common questions?

When can you resume exercise? What about vigorous exercise?

_____

_____

Are there any limitations to the type of exercises you can do? When can you get into a pool?

_____

_____

Which compression garments (if any) should you wear and when should you switch into a smaller sized garment? Is there any medical reason you shouldn't wear a garment?

_____

_____

When can you start taking supplements again after surgery?

_____

_____

When will your drains or stitches be removed? What should you do if fluid suddenly stops draining?

_____

_____

Do you have any dissolvable stitches? What should you do if your incision opens up?

_____

_____

Are you allowed to use a cool compress or heat on the surgical area?

_____

_____

When are you allowed to get acupuncture?

_____

_____

What are the warning signs that you may have an infection or seroma? What should you do if you suspect you have an infection or seroma?

_____

_____

How long will you feel numbness?

_____

_____

How long is your recovery? This is tricky, because there are so many definitions of "recovery". Here are some sample questions: When can you return to work? When will you begin to feel good in clothes? How long until you can be in a friend's wedding, with all the photos and partying? How long until you can feel good in a bathing suit on the beach? How long until you can go on a week-long sightseeing vacation with lots of walking?

_____

_____

How can you contact your surgeon's office with questions at night or on weekends?

_____

_____

Other questions you want to ask your surgeon at your follow-up visit:

_____

_____

_____

Bottom line: following doctor's orders is key to your recovery!

"Create your own style. Let it be unique for yourself and yet identifiable for others." — Anna Wintour

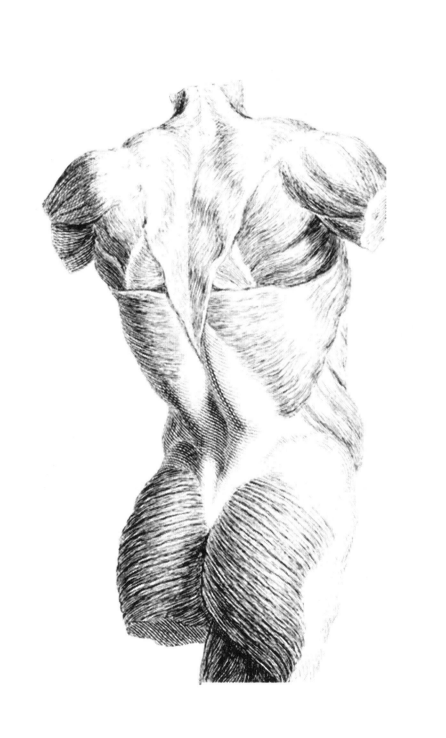

CHAPTER 3
REDUCING SWELLING

Dealing with swelling was the worst part of recovering from my facial surgeries. It's a constant negative reminder of the surgery; it makes it harder to move and can feel heavy or tight. You might feel embarrassed to go out in public if you have had a facelift. Swelling after liposuction is also extremely discouraging for many of my clients. They paid good money to change their figure and now they can barely fit into clothes that used to be comfortable!

It is completely natural for your body to have swelling after surgery. In his book A Patient's Guide to Liposuction, Dr. Schafer says "swelling is caused by an accumulation of excess fluid in the treated tissue" (2001). Swelling is normal, but if you are a proactive person who wants to get back to your normal life, there's no reason to just wait patiently until it subsides on its own.

Is My Swelling Getting Worse?

Do you feel like your swelling after liposuction is increasing day by day in the first week after surgery? It's not all in your head! In fact, in the book *Bodysculpture: Plastic Surgery of the Body for Men and Women*, Dr. Engler says after liposuction, "maximum swelling and bruising—and therefore discomfort—may not occur until 1–3 days after the surgery. When bruising starts out relatively deep (as after a liposuction), it may take longer to peak, e.g., 5–10 days" (2000). In the study "Unfavourable Outcomes of Liposuction and Their Management," published in the Indian Journal of Plastic Surgery, Dixit and Wagh (2013) reviewed the cases of over six hundred liposuction procedures and found that "swelling will be apparent within 24–48 [hours] after the procedure and continues to mildly increase for the first 10–14 days."

Help! I'm STILL Swollen!

Do you feel like some parts of your body are staying swollen longer than others? It may be true! In the article "A Journey Through Liposuction and Liposculture: Review" published in the Annals of Medicine & Surgery, Bellini et al. found that edema "in some venous areas such as ankles and calves may persist for six months or a year" (2017).

How Can I Get Rid of Swelling after Surgery?

Once surgical incisions have closed, the body removes swelling through the lymphatic system. It's completely okay to not know much about this system of the body— we probably weren't taught about it in high school physiology class. The lymphatic system is our body's recycling system—a network of vessels that transports water, fat molecules, proteins and waste products from the interstitial fluid around our cells back to the heart. Specifically, "lymph vessels participate in the formation of lymph from the interstitial fluid and conduct lymph to the venous system" (Foldi & Foldi, 2012, 5). It is also part of our immune system. Lymphatic fluid is filtered through the lymph nodes, and when tissue is damaged and vessels leading to lymph nodes are cut or damaged during surgery, short-term swelling can occur.

There are several ways to reduce swelling, including:

- Manual Lymphatic Drainage (MLD) massage
- Exercise and joint movement
- Diaphragmatic (belly) breathing
- External compression
- Kinesiology Taping
- Vibration
- Cooling treatments that reduce blood flow through vasoconstriction

Let's look at each of these techniques in more depth.

Manual Lymphatic Drainage (MLD) Massage

What is Manual Lymphatic Drainage? There is a lot of confusion on social media. Many massage therapists are pushing fluid out of open incisions and calling it manual lymphatic drainage. It is done manually, and it is drainage, but the fluid is not going through the interstitium and not the lymphatic system, so it's not proper Manual Lymphatic Drainage. I consider it more like a milking stroke. Some surgeons use a similar milking stroke to reduce swelling immediately after surgery in the operating room. Pushing fluid out of incisions is beneficial and can reduce swelling while incisions are still open. If you have open incisions, your surgeon will give you guidance on how to keep them safe from infection.

So, what can you do to reduce swelling after your drains are removed or your incisions are closed? This is when Manual Lymphatic Drainage is helpful.

Manual Lymphatic Drainage is a gentle skin stretching massage technique that encourages swelling to move into our body's lymphatic system. The skin stretch is what makes it most effective—it is not a milking, rubbing or sliding type of massage. According to "Nonoperative Treatment of Lymphedema," published in *Seminars in Plastic Surgery*, "manual lymph drainage is a technique used to increase the lymphatic fluid transport rate, develop new routes for lymphatic drainage from congested areas to adjacent nonedematous regions, increase the activity of macrophages to breakdown protein deposits, and mechanically break up fibrotic tissue. It is indicated in patients with significant pitting edema of the extremity, trunk, or chest wall, with fibrotic or sclerotic tissue changes, and in those with significant symptoms including heaviness or tightness" (Schaverien, Moeller & Cleveland, 2018). If you feel heavy or tight, try Manual Lymphatic Drainage.

The lymphatic system will keep on working hard to remove swelling as best it can for some time after the massage. Swelling leaves the body in the urine. I recommend at least two one-hour sessions per week for as long as swelling feels uncomfortable. Some clients only want a few weeks of treatment and others receive Manual Lymphatic Drainage regularly for a few months to achieve optimal results.

My top tips for clients:

- Put your compression garment on as soon as possible after the MLD treatment.
- Please drink plenty of water! Water is essential for your body. Reducing water intake will NOT reduce swelling.
- You may urinate more (it's how swelling leaves the body) and your urine might smell or feel different.
- You may become less constipated as a result of the abdominal work that is part of your treatment.
- Manual Lymphatic Drainage is not a silver bullet or a quick fix. Your swelling will not be completely resolved in only one or two sessions.

What is the research behind using Manual Lymphatic Drainage to reduce swelling?

Doctors Renato Saltz and Bianca Ohana studied 183

patients who had undergone an endoscopic midface lift. In "Postoperative Instructions for Patients," published in *Aesthetic Surgery Journal*, Saltz and Ohana recommend elevating the head, using cold compresses over the eyes, and "lymphatic drainage massage 72 hours postoperatively, once or twice during the first week, then 2–3 times a week" (2012).

Lymphatic massage has a positive impact after orthopedic surgery as well. In the study "Randomized Trial Investigating the Efficacy of Manual Lymphatic Drainage to Improve Early Outcome After Total Knee Arthroplasty" published in the Archives of Physical Medicine and Rehabilitation, Ebert et al. found that performing a half hour of manual lymphatic drainage massage on days 2, 3 and 4 after a total knee arthroplasty "appears to improve active knee flexion up to 6 weeks postsurgery." Why is this important? Because "restricted postoperative knee [range of motion] remains one of the most frequent postoperative complications and indicators for patient dissatisfaction" (2013).

Olesen & Olesen share that their patients find Manual Lymphatic Drainage massage "not only relaxes them but also contributes significantly to their recovery" and that "some surgeons recommend one session before surgery as well as after surgery" while "other surgeons encourage only postsurgery appointments" (2005).

This technique has a long history! People have used Manual Lymphatic Drainage to heal from Plastic Surgery for over 20 years. In the presentation "Manual Lymphatic Drainage Therapy: An Integral Component of Postoperative Care in Plastic Surgery Patients," given at the first annual conference of the American Society of Lymphology, Dr. Casas and Dr. DePoli (1999) found that when clients recovering from surgery (liposuction of the abdomen, buttocks, hips or thighs, abdominoplasty/tummy tuck, or facelift) were treated with Manual Lymphatic Drainage massage and deep tissue massage 1–2 times per week for the first 3–6 weeks following their operation, with deep tissue massage given as subcutaneous fibrosis developed, they recovered faster. Fibrosis is the thickening or scarring of connective tissue in the body. We'll talk more about fibrosis in the Improving Scars and Fibrosis chapter.

How fast is faster?

Casas and DePoli (1999) stated that without any postoperative decongestive therapy "we see complete resolution of postoperative edema and fibrosis in this group between 9 months to 18 months following surgery. In the ten groups listed above who underwent MLD and Deep Tissue Massage, postoperative swelling and fibrosis resolved within 6 weeks to 3 months, thereby shortening recovery significantly."

When we are healthy, our bodies use movement and muscle contractions to move lymphatic fluid. Manual Lymphatic Drainage massage can help move lymphatic fluid when clients are prohibited from engaging in vigorous exercise in the first weeks after surgery. Guenter Klose, one of my teachers and an expert in the treatment of lymphedema, says "postsurgical clients who can benefit from manual lymph drainage include those recovering from cosmetic surgeries such as face-lifts, breast augmentation, and liposuction and orthopedic surgeries such as joint repair or replacement. Manual lymph drainage effectively reduces swelling even before appropriate muscle movement and function can be restored" (2014). Often, a surgeon will only allow very light exercise in the weeks after surgery. Manual Lymphatic Drainage massage can help reduce swelling before patients are allowed to use exercise and joint movement to help their lymphatic system.

Exercise and Joint Movement

Exercising can be very gentle and still effective for boosting lymphatic flow after liposuction. You don't need to break a sweat. Just flexing and extending your joints and muscles, especially your diaphragm and calf muscles, helps move lymphatic fluid through your system.

Always check with your surgeon before starting any new type of exercise. Olesen & Olesen are right when they say "you need to expect limits on your normal activities and exercise during your recovery" (2005). On their website, the American Society for Aesthetic Plastic Surgery (ASAPS) cautions that liposuction clients should "avoid strenuous exercise for four to six weeks because it can trigger unnecessary fluid retention in the treated areas."

- Going for a walk can be a gentle form of exercise and still very effective for increasing lymphatic flow.
- If you have leg or foot swelling, try leg range of motion exercises. Try to perform up to one minute of ankle pumps (flexion and extension) once or twice per hour when you are awake—it may increase blood flow for up to 30 minutes.

Too much exercise too soon can increase swelling, even if the "exercise" is just walking around and shopping for a few hours.

Many people experience numbness after surgery, which means you may not know if you are overexerting yourself. Rest assured, numbness is totally normal. In the book *Liposuction Principles and Practice*, Melvin A. Shiffman, MD, says "decreased sensation or sensory loss may occur but is almost always temporary" (2006, 337).

Even after you are allowed to resume exercise, still be sure to ask your doctor if vigorous stretches are right for you. There is more information on exercising after surgery later in the book.

Diaphragmatic (Belly) Breathing

Belly breathing activates the diaphragm, which boosts our body's lymphatic flow. Indeed, Foldi and Foldi say lymphatic flow is "clearly dependent upon respiration" (2012, 551).

Too many of us take shallow breaths. If you have any small children or babies in your life, take a moment to watch them breathe. They will most likely move their tummies as they breathe. Sometime long ago, when we were kids, maybe somebody made fun of the way we breathed or we squeezed ourselves into constricting clothes and we stopped belly breathing. Did you know that 83% of people with anxiety have breath dysfunction (Courtney, 2009)? If you have anxiety, it might be another great reason to give belly breathing a try.

Do you belly breathe?

Test yourself now by taking a breath with your hand placed over your belly button. Does your belly push out or does it remain motionless or get sucked in as you inhale? That's the difference between belly breathing and shallow breathing.

Let's practice belly breathing now.

Place your hands along the bottom of your ribcage, near your belly button. If you tend to get a tense jaw, try putting the tip of your tongue at the roof of your mouth to relax your jaw. Take a deep breath through your nose and allow your abdomen to expand. Can you feel your rib cage widen and your tummy push out? Exhale completely. This is belly or diaphragmatic breathing.

A common body pose that makes us instantly think of

being relaxed can actually help you to practice belly breathing! Try it by lying on your back, stretching your arms overhead, then clasping your hands together behind your head. You look relaxed and you are also cueing your body to use your abdomen to breathe.

If you can't get the hang of it, try watching this video by Dr. Belisa Vranich to learn more about breathing: https://youtu.be/ysYO69Oxdhc

External Compression

If you had liposuction or a tummy tuck, your plastic surgeon may have given you a compression garment. Wearing the garment as prescribed will help decrease swelling by providing external resistance, which helps limit further swelling and encourages the lymphatic system to draw excess fluid away from your surgical area.

Many of my plastic surgery clients come to their first visit already wearing compression garments prescribed by their surgeon. Compression garments are more than just a super-expensive pair of tights. Wearing a correctly fitted garment with the proper level of compression is an important part of recovery.
I know, I know. Compression is expensive and a pain to wear. If you need some convincing, let's see what plastic surgery experts recommend to their own patients.

On its website, ASAPS recommends that liposuction patients "wear a compression garment over the treated areas for four to six weeks to control swelling and promote skin contraction." They also tell clients recovering from tummy tucks that doing so "reduces the likelihood of loose or sagging skin after an abdominoplasty. The compression garment also helps to control swelling, resulting in a shorter recovery period" (n.d.b.).

Dixit and Wagh say "some of the methods that are commonly employed to minimise post-operative oedema [swelling, or edema] are: applying an optimum compressive garment immediately after surgery... providing manual lymphatic drainage in the early post-operative period. In our experience gentle liposuctioning, an optimum compressive garment and early lymphatic drainage massage helps to accelerate the clearance of oedema" (2013).

Schafer says "compression garments are essential to recovery after liposuction. They apply pressure to the treated area to keep the tissue from shifting as the patient moves," they "help control pain and swelling" and "a foam insert may be used under the garment to reduce the possibility of blood or other fluids collecting (and decrease bruising)" (2011).

Shiffman says "persistent edema in the area of liposuction can be distressing to the patient. This may be due to excessive trauma to the tissues but liposuction is a traumatic procedure causing so called internal burnlike injury. Proper compression is usually the key for prevention" (2006, 334).

Miami, Florida, is a hotbed for plastic surgery. I have clients who travel to Miami for their surgery and fly back home to San Diego to recuperate. If you want to have a Miami-style surgery result, you need to do what the ladies in Miami do—wear your compression garment and lipo foam and invest in lymphatic massages. (If you are traveling for plastic surgery, I highly recommend you read Massage Therapist Marian Sotelo-Paz's book *Before & After: A Guide for Cosmetic Surgery* for tips on how to book transportation and recovery care).

Foam is a Compression Garment's Best Friend

Why use foam? I first experienced the practice of using a combination of foam and compression for reducing edema in my training as a Certified Lymphedema Therapist. Foam pads placed underneath your compression garment will put constant, gentle pressure on any patches of swelling on the torso, arms, and legs, encouraging the extra fluid to be reabsorbed. Read more about foam in Chapter 5.

Bottom Line: A layer of foam will help evenly distribute compression, making the compression garment more effective at reducing swelling and keeping it out of the area.

Please read this if you are considering using Reston foam after surgery: https://multimedia.3m.com/mws/media/820830/common-questions-reston-self-adhering-foam-products.pdf.

What if you no longer need a lot of compression?

Micromassage and light compression garments are another option for chronic edema. My colleagues have seen clients who have a lipedema diagnosis and are suffering with chronic swelling achieve a reduction in these symptoms by using a micromassage compression garment next to their skin. Several garments on the market provide a moderate level of compression. **Bioflect®**, **CzSalus®** and **Solidea®** are three brands. This may be a good option if you have chronic swelling and are no longer wearing your postsurgical compression garment, or feel you need a little more compression than your current garment provides. If you feel ill or swell more when wearing the micromassage compression, stop wearing it.

What about those socks you were given after surgery?

Some surgeons ask their patients to wear anti-embolism stockings. Sometimes called T.E.D. hose, which is short for Thrombo-Embolic Deterrent, these are a pair of socks with light compression used to reduce the risk of a blood clot. These garments are designed to work when you are horizontal—lying down in bed or on the couch. Once you can stand and walk around easily, you'll have to switch into a stronger pair of compression socks if you need to reduce swelling in your legs and feet.

What is Bimodal Compression?

Some plastic surgeons leave liposuction incisions open to allow the swelling to leave the body faster than if the incisions were closed immediately after surgery. If you have open incisions, your surgeon may use Bimodal Compression, which is the "sequential use of two different stages of post-liposuction compression" (Kassardjian, n.d.).

Getting Compression Right

Talk to your surgeon if you are experiencing any of the following:

- **Too-tight compression garment.** Often, a few sessions of lymphatic massage will reduce swelling enough to make the garment more comfortable. If you are experiencing pain, lightheadedness or dizziness when wearing compression garments, work with your surgeon to find a level of compression and/or a garment that is right for you. You can also work with a Certified Lymphedema Therapist to figure out additional options for compression.

- **Too-loose compression garment.** Many of my clients get good results from switching to a compression garment in a smaller size a few weeks to a month after their operation. Sizing down is a time of celebration! It means the lymphatic system is working to reduce swelling and the body is healing.

- **Compression garment that bunches or leaves lines in the skin.** Make sure that your garment doesn't have any wrinkles or bunched areas while you are wearing it during the day. Padding or foam may also help. Wrinkles and bunching may cause the skin underneath to become wavy or fibrotic. Double-check the smoothness of the garment when driving and sitting. Shiffman says "following liposuction, folds in the garment can result in indentations and subcutaneous fibrosis. The garment should be checked on the first postoperative day and the patient informed of how to prevent or limit folds in the garment (especially an abdominal binder)" (2006, 335).

- **Foam pieces that don't provide even compression around the torso.** You may need to switch or customize your foam pieces.

Care for your garments! Wash them according to the instructions on the tag. Here are some tips on taking care of your post-surgical garments:

Bonito & Co.® garments "cannot be machine-washed and machine dried. Please hand wash (with a gentle detergent) and air dry (about 5 hours to dry) your garment, and when dry, please place it into the pouch you received it in, and place it into the refrigerator for 20–30 min, which allows the fibers of the very high-end material to reconstitute and recompress, so you receive the exact same compression ratio, as when it was new, and ultimate compression every time you wear your garment" (FAQ, 2019).

ClearPoint Medical® garments should be "hand wash in cold water using a mild detergent cold water rinse and hang dry" The don't recommend machine washing or drying or using bleach. The company website recommends that you "remove stains by rubbing baking soda, an environmentally friendly compound, on the area(s). Baking soda can also be used as an alternative to detergent" (Frequently Asked Questions, n.d.).

Contemporary Design® garments recommends that you "hand wash your compression garment in lukewarm water with a mild detergent and then air dry. Please do not dry your garment in a gas or electric dryer, for it may ruin the garment. Drip dry, do not wring out. Delicate or synthetic fabrics tend to dry quite quickly. To remove bloodstains, simply soak your garment in a basin of cool water mixed with a ¼ cup of peroxide" (How to Videos & Care, n.d.)

Design Veronique® recommends that their garments have "cold water washing and line drying.
For stain removal, soak the product in 2 to 3 gallons of cold water with ¼ cup of peroxide for 15 minutes, and follow recommended care instructions" (The Fitting Room, n.d.).

HK Surgical® garments should be machine washed and laid flat to dry.

Isavela® compression garments should be "hand-wash in cold water using a mild fabric wash. Do not use bleach. Rinse thoroughly in cold water and drip dry." Remove stains by soaking the garment in "2 to 3 gallons of cold water and 1/2 cup of peroxide for 30 minutes" (Direction Of Use And Care, n.d.).

Jobst® Plastic Surgery Girdles can be hand washed or machine washed in a mesh laundry bag. The company recommends using warm water, a mild soap or detergent and discourages the use of fabric softeners (Wear & Care, n.d.).

Leonisa® garment instructions are: hand wash cold, do not tumble dry, do not use bleach, use a soft detergent.

Marena® Compression Garments are machine wash gentle and tumble dry low (Care Instructions, n.d.).

Medical Z® garments should be washed at 30 degrees celsius and be machine dried.

Rainey Recovery Wear® garments should be washed in cold water with mild detergent, regular cycle and tumble dry with no heat.

Wear Ease® garments should be laundered "according to the care tag attached to the garment. For best results, wash in a lingerie bag. Do not use chlorine bleach or fabric softener. Tumble dry low or hang to dry" (Garment Care, 2017).

Micro-massage Garments:

Bioflect® FIR Therapy garments should be hand washed with mild detergent and laid flat to dry. Garments are also machine washable on the delicate cycle. Do not use fabric softener or dry clean (General Product Information & FAQs, n.d.)

CzSalus® polyamide microfiber garments can be turned inside-out and machine washed at a lower temperature.

Solidea® garments can be hand-washed using a mild detergent. Gently squeeze out excess water (do not wring) and lay flat to dry. The garment can also be machine-washed in a lingerie bag with warm water on the delicate cycle and dried at a low temperature setting. They do not recommend using bleach, fabric softener or other laundry additives (Garment Care, n.d.).

More Compression Garment Tips

Wash your compression garment daily. If you need a shower, so does your garment.

Air drying is good, but if the tag says that you can machine dry the garment, put your compression garment in the dryer for a few minutes, too. It will help the garment keep its shape.

Sun breaks down elastic, so keep compression garments out of the sun as much as possible.

Heavy, greasy lotions break down a garment's elastic. Do keep your skin hydrated and moisturize your body with a low-pH lotion, but let it fully absorb into your skin before putting on your garment.

If it's hard to sit down to pee in your garment, consider trying a urination funnel. They are made of a flexible material and shaped to allow you to urinate while standing. This is especially useful after a breast augmentation surgery if you have difficulty standing from a seated position.

If your legs start developing blisters in the garment, please ask your physician to check you for arterial disease.

If your compression garment has an opening for you to go to the bathroom, make sure that skin from your thighs remains fully inside the garment, so that your legs benefit from the compression of the garment.

If you are having a difficult time putting on your garment, the "My FAJA doesn't fit!?!?!" video has some tips: https://youtu.be/7kMBiGfE7iE. This video from Curvy Gyals titled "Curvy Gyals- How To Put On Our St. Azar Traditional Faja" may also be helpful: https://youtu.be/34jkAFe2RKU.

Reduce Swelling When You Travel

Be sure to wear your compression garments when you are flying. In the research article "The Effect of Compression Stocking on Leg Edema and Discomfort During a 3-hour Flight: A Randomized Controlled Trial" published in the European Journal of Internal Medicine, Olsen et. al (2019) found "compression stockings reduced edema formation in young healthy passengers during a three-hour flight." Many of my post-plastic surgery clients must travel for their careers. While traveling, it's a good idea to wear compression garments as much as possible, walk around during the flight or at rest stops if traveling by car, and book extra lymphatic drainage massage sessions after the trip to reduce swelling.

Qantas airline offers a video of stretching exercises you can do in an airplane at https://youtu.be/Gv7enzl7Yq8. A simple tip is to perform one minute of ankle pumps (flexion and extension) once or twice per hour when you are awake on the flight — it may increase blood flow for up to thirty minutes.

Water Helps Reduce Swelling

Water pressure is another form of external compression. Spending time in the water helps to reduce swelling. The Bone, Muscle and Joint team at the Cleveland Clinic recommend exercises that move the ankle and knee joints, like walking and swimming, to reduce swelling (Cleveland Clinic, 2016). The pressure of the water on the lower body when standing in a pool or other body of water is also effective for reducing swelling, so water aerobics is another great option.

How do you know it's working? You'll want to pee! Be sure to ask your doctor first before getting into the pool or ocean. You will want to wait until scars are closed and healing well.

Help! I'm Swollen Down There!

Do you have swelling in your private parts right after surgery? Shiffman says "labial and scrotal edema is common but temporary" (2006, 99). Dixit and Wagh (2013) say "we have also observed a unique seroma-like presentation when the fluid gravitates to the scrotum or labia following abdominal, especially pubic fat liposuction. In our experience... it usually settles over 10 days to 2 weeks. We have managed to largely prevent this problem by restricting excessive mobility for the first 3 days after surgery and having the patients wear a snug fitting undergarment over the compression garment."

According to women's health physiotherapist Michelle Lyons, "orgasm can be a great way to decrease stagnation and improve circulation in the pelvis, as the female orgasm is a series of rhythmic contractions of the pelvic floor muscles, 0.7 seconds apart." She points out that "orgasm will also promote happy hormones like dopamine, oxytocin and serotonin and keep cortisol levels down—great for parasympathetic functionality, wound healing and immune resilience."

Lyons shares that "the other key driver of success would be avoiding constipation—so hydration, a diet rich in vegetables and fruit and movement—a 20 minute daily walk has been shown to be effective—and would generally be beneficial for surgical recovery as well."

Ask your surgeon when it is okay to have sex, either with yourself and with another person. You can find free resources on pelvic floor health and reducing constipation at Lyons' website https://celebratemuliebrity.com.

Compression may also help. You can purchase a special foam piece designed to help women with genital lymphedema if you are concerned about genital swelling. Learn more about the garment at https://youtu.be/_3RI-A3Gwfs.

Kinesiology Taping

Many lymphedema therapists, massage therapists, physical therapists and athletic trainers use kinesiology tape to reduce swelling in their clients. The theory behind using kinesiology tape to reduce swelling is that the tape gently lifts the skin, changing the interstitial pressure and encouraging lymphatic vessels to take more fluid back to the heart. The key to effective lymphatic kinesiology taping is to put absolutely no stretch on the tape as it is applied.

Kinesiology taping has been proven to work after orthopedic surgery. In the study, "The effectiveness of **Kinesio Taping**® after total knee replacement in early postoperative rehabilitation period. A randomized clinical trial," published in the *European Journal of Physical and Rehabilitation Medicine*, Donec and Kriščiūnas found the "Kinesio taping® technique, applied during the study, appeared to be beneficial for reducing postoperative pain, edema, improving knee extension in early postoperative rehabilitation period" (2014).

Ask your plastic surgeon if using kinesiology tape to reduce swelling is right for you. It may be a good option, even if you are wearing a compression garment over your area of swelling. Be sure to do a patch test in advance to make sure you have no sensitivity to the tape.

It might be difficult to remove kinesiology tape if you have sensitive skin or if the tape has been pulled too tight. Protect your skin by saturating the taped area with a cotton ball soaked with olive oil before removing it. Wait a few minutes, then resaturate the area with more olive oil as you remove the tape. A fellow Certified Lymphedema Therapist shared another tip with me: applying a thin coat of magnesium hydroxide (**Milk of Magnesia**®) and letting it dry before applying kinesiology tape may reduce skin sensitivity.

Clare Anvar and I were both speakers at the 2019 MLD UK Conference in Great Britain and I had the opportunity to see some of her post-plastic surgery taping techniques in person. For more information on kinesiology taping after plastic surgery, read her article "On Tape" at http://media.wix.com/ugd/1e5d09_2155c62b8ba245c181ed4379bb016c1c.pdf.

Kenzo Kase also has an excellent guide for practitioners titled *Kinesio Taping for Lymphoedema and Chronic Swelling*.

Vibration

Deep Oscillation is one of several treatments that use vibration to reduce edema. In the article "Safety and Effectiveness of Vibration Massage by Deep Oscillations: A Prospective Observational Study," published in *Evidence Based Complementary and Alternative Medicine*, Kraft et al. say "deep oscillation massage is used to stimulate the absorption of edema, to reduce pain, and to alleviate wound healing as well as for its anti-inflammatory and antifibrous effects." A deep oscillation machine creates "a pulsating electrostatic field of low intensity and frequency ... between the manual applicator and the patients' tissue" which affects "skin, subcutaneous tissue, muscles, blood vessels and lymphatic vessels, and presumably an increased local vascular circulation" (2013). A large majority of the therapists at the MLD UK conference I attended in 2019 use deep oscillation on their patients, but it's not as widely used in the US.

Other vibration therapies that may reduce edema include gently bouncing on a rebounder and using a whole-body vibration machine. Ask your plastic surgeon if using vibration is right for you. They may want to limit these types of therapies immediately after surgery.

Cooling Treatments

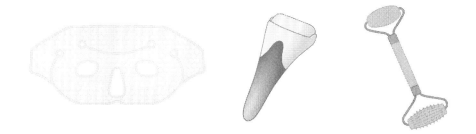

Cooling techniques encourage vasoconstriction and are a good way to reduce pain, inflammation and swelling temporarily. Cooling can also be used for everyday swelling, especially the morning after a fun night out! Make sure to ask your plastic surgeon if it is okay to use cooling techniques on your face and body before trying these products. I'd recommend NOT using cooling techniques on the affected area if you have had a fat transfer. To reduce the risk of frostbite, please don't use cooling treatments on areas of skin that still feel numb after surgery.

- **Face Mask:** I use a plastic face mask that can be kept in the refrigerator to reduce puffiness in my eyes and face.
- **Face Roller:** Back in 2015, all the beauty magazines and bloggers discovered face rollers! They still work to reduce puffiness in the face. I store my face rollers in the freezer. Use the lymphatic diagram of the face to roll in the direction of lymphatic drainage.
- **Sheet Mask:** A word of caution about using sheet masks. One popular ingredient for reducing

inflammation is caffeine. Topically applied caffeine has a strong reputation for reducing swelling, but a study published in the July 2014 International Wound Journal found that caffeine may negatively affect wound healing (Ojeh et al., 2016). Don't worry, this doesn't mean you can't drink coffee. My advice: ask your plastic surgeon if it's okay to use caffeine near your incision area.

- **Jade Roller:** When used correctly according to the lymphatic drainage diagram, jade rollers can help boost lymphatic drainage. Jade is cooling and can be stored in the refrigerator or freezer.

- **Cool Compresses:** The American Society for Aesthetic Plastic Surgery (ASAPS) recommends that clients recovering from a facelift "apply cool (not cold) compresses to your eyes… Soak soft, white washcloths or gauze squares in ice water and wring out well. Apply directly to the eyes, but not to the cheeks or neck. Do not apply any pressure. Apply cool compresses for no longer than twenty-minute intervals" (Facelift, 2018).

More Ways to Reduce Swelling

What to Eat To Reduce Swelling

It's important to make sure you're getting enough protein, vitamins and minerals in your diet to support the healing process.

Dixit and Wagh (2013) say "persistent oedema can also be related to pre-operative anaemia, reduced serum proteins and kidney malfunction all [of] which are a contraindication to surgery." Make sure you are getting enough iron and protein in your diet. Some supplements, including turmeric, may inhibit your body's ability to absorb iron (Smith & Ashar, 2019).

In the article "Factors That Impair Wound Healing," published in the *Journal of the American College of Clinical Wound Specialists*, Anderson and Hamm say "insufficient protein intake can be assessed utilizing hematological markers such as albumin and pre-albumin or total lymphocyte count. Other diagnostic tools, namely the Rainey MacDonald nutritional index (RMNI) or the Mini-nutritional assessment (MNA), are useful in assessing risk or presence of protein malnutrition" (2014).

If you are concerned about your diet, discuss it with your surgeon, primary care physician, or dietician to make sure you are getting the nutrition you need.

How to Sleep to Reduce Swelling

Many plastic surgeons recommend their patients sleep with their head elevated on two or three pillows for a few weeks after facelift surgery. Elevating the head uses gravity to help drain the post-surgical swelling through the lymphatic system. Yes, your neck is likely to feel stiff from sleeping like that, but it's worth it. ASAPS recommends that while recovering from a facelift you "sleep with your head elevated forty degrees for two weeks; an additional pillow or two under your mattress may help, if necessary" (Facelift, 2018).

How can you make sure you're not sleeping on your side? In his book *Straight Talk About Cosmetic Surgery*, Dr. Arthur W. Perry recommends his facelift clients also use a "U-shaped travel pillow or pillow with arms" to remind them not to turn over while sleeping. Alternately, patients can try sleeping in a recliner (2007). Another option is to place pillows underneath your arms on either side of your torso to reduce your ability to roll over.

Dry Brushing

Dry brushing involves brushing the skin with a specific type of brush in order to engage the lymphatic system. Does it work? What are some tips to have the best results? The trouble is that most of what I read online are the exact same "rules" with no explanation of where they came from or if they have any backing in science.

Let's tackle the science part first. I found three articles that consult medical experts. The Cleveland Clinic recommends dry brushing to promote lymph flow and drainage (Starkey, 2015). The *New York Times* reports Dr. Tina S. Alster, a clinical professor of dermatology at Georgetown University Medical Center, finds dry brushing helps the lymphatic system "work better" (Saint Louis, 2010).

My keys to dry brushing are using a brush that is soft and caring for the integrity of the skin, especially if the immune system is compromised. The stroke should not just pet or glide across the skin. We have to move and stretch the skin in order to open up the initial lymphatic vessels and reduce swelling.

My Top 5 Tips on How to Dry Brush

- If you use natural bristles, make sure your dry brush has never been used (gotten wet) in the shower or bath. Keep a separate one just for brushing
- If you are cautious of using natural bristles because of the potential for skin damage, use a soft rubbery pet hairbrush for dry brushing
- Brush in strokes that follow the pathway of the lymphatic system
- Brush before showering or first thing in the morning, when skin is dry
- Don't brush too much! Stop before skin becomes sensitive or turns red
- Moisturize after you dry brush (or after the post-brushing shower)

If you want to try dry brushing, use the following diagram:

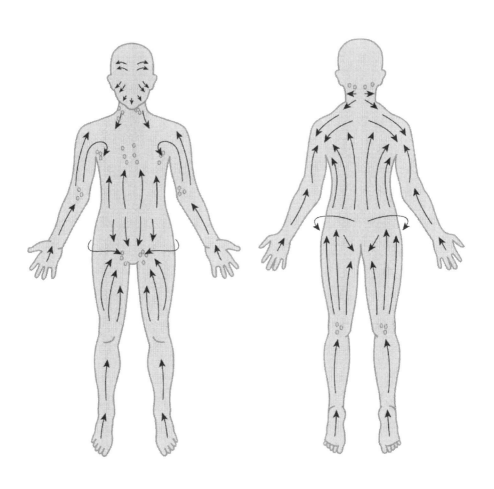

Ask your surgeon for an okay before trying dry brushing, and avoid brushing over your incisions. You can often brush all other areas of your body, only avoiding the skin around the surgical area.

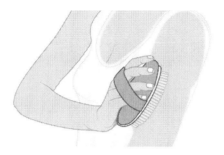

What are some ways you have healed your swelling in the past? Did your parents or grandparents have a home remedy that worked? Write down that advice here:

_____

_____

A Final Note on Swelling

There are some forms of swelling that manual lymphatic drainage and exercise cannot help. If only one leg or arm is swollen and the swelling came on suddenly, let your doctor know immediately. It may be a blood clot. If a limb is swollen because of infection, a blood clot, heart failure or kidney failure, lymphatic massage is not allowed.

"The self is not something one finds; it is something one creates." — George Bernard Shaw

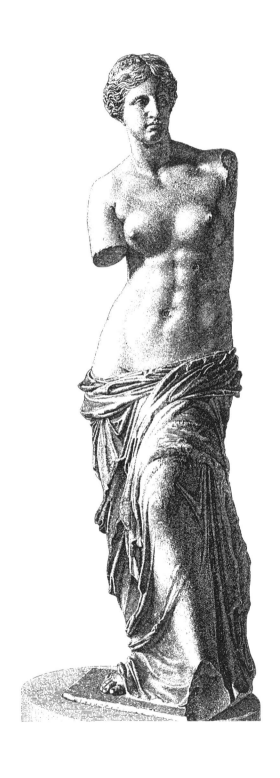

CHAPTER 4
REDUCING BRUISING

After my skiing accident, my boss actually sent me home to sit on my couch for a few days before my surgery because the bruising on my face was so hideous. Even when bruising doesn't hurt that much, just seeing our bodies all black and blue sets off little alarm bells in our head. We don't want to look at ourselves and don't want anyone else to see us either.

We all bruise, but what exactly is happening when we get a bruise? Schafer says "bruising is the result of blood pooling into subcutaneous tissue under the skin or in mucous membranes" (2001). Olesen and Olesen say "as the blood is absorbed by the body, the color of the bruise gradually changes from purplish to red to greenish and then to yellow" (2005). How much you will bruise after surgery depends partly on your individual body. Dixit and Wagh found that severe bruising was usually related to chronic smoking or the use of blood thinners (2013). I have seen extensive bruising and little to no bruising on different clients after the same type of operation.

How can we help bruises heal faster?

Shiffman says "compression over the areas of liposuctioning will help to limit bruising. This includes the use of garments, stretch tape, and foam dressings (polyurethane pads)" (2006, 333).

Kinesiology taping can quite dramatically reduce the appearance of bruises. The tape seems to work by lifting the skin away from the body, which encourages circulation.

Doctors Michael Hamman and Mitchel Goldman share information on how to reduce bruising in the article "Minimizing Bruising Following Fillers and Other Cosmetic Injectables" published in the *Journal of Clinical and Aesthetic Dermatology*. Hamman & Goldman recommend "if aspirin is not medically necessary, it should be held for one week prior to any injectable procedure. The patient should also avoid the use of nonsteroidal anti-inflammatory medications for five days prior to any procedures." They also say "high-dose vitamin E, ginkgo biloba, and garlic have case reports and studies demonstrating increased bleeding and/or bruising. Many physicians recommend that patients stop taking these two weeks prior to any procedure" (2013).

Several plastic surgeons I know recommend arnica montana to help with pain and bruising after surgery. Other surgeons don't want their patients to use anything on the skin. I sometimes use arnica montana topically in my massage studio with clients.

Some of my clients eat more pineapple after their surgery because raw pineapple contains bromelain. In the article "Nutritional Support for Wound Healing," MacKay and Miller say "750–1,000 mg bromelain post-operatively may reduce edema, bruising, pain, and healing time following trauma and surgical procedures" (2003).

Make sure you have a conversation with your surgeon before you start or stop taking any medications or supplements.

What are some ways you have healed your bruises in the past? Did your parents or grandparents have a home remedy that worked? Write that advice here:

_____

_____

"One should either be a work of art, or wear a work of art."
— Oscar Wilde

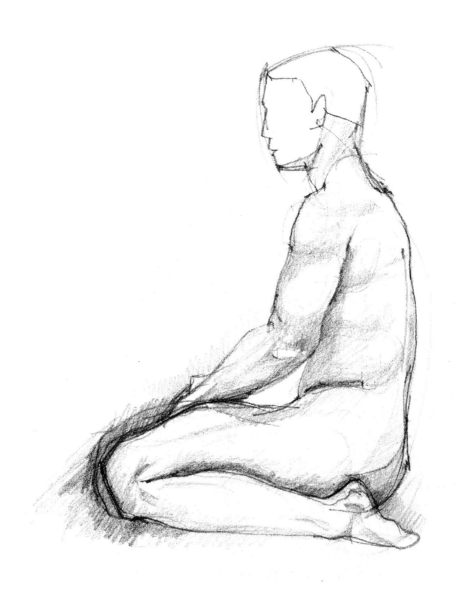

CHAPTER 5

IMPROVING SCARS AND FIBROSIS

Let's focus on scars first, then talk about fibrosis after liposuction. I was lucky that my facial reconstructive surgery didn't leave any scars on my skin (one of the incisions was in my lower eyelid and the other was inside my mouth), but my Mohs surgery for skin cancer on my face left a scar that was initially very shocking and upsetting to me. Happily, that scar has now faded. I used scar strips and laser treatment in the months after my surgery to reduce its color and prominence.

One question I often hear from my clients is: When will my scar fade? Engler says "scars normally fade quite acceptably (typically within several months, although it can take up to one or two years for a scar to mature completely), but there is no guarantee that they will do so. Different types of skin heal differently. In general, thicker skin heals less well (i.e., leaves worse scars) than thinner skin" (2000).

Lasers and Scars

If you are feeling nervous and self-conscious about your scars, have a chat with your surgeon or dermatologist early in in your recovery and make a plan for treating your scars.

What kinds of treatments can help scars? In the book Instant Beauty, Dr. Steven H. Dayan says "we've learned from doing laser treatments to remove wrinkles that we can influence the way collagen remodels itself following a laser treatment. Therefore, using this same philosophy, I now address scars very early in with a series of ablative erbium laser treatments" (2007).

In the review article "Advances in the Treatment of Traumatic Scars with Laser, Intense Pulsed Light, Radiofrequency, and Ultrasound" published in *Burns & Trauma*, Fu et al. say "the management for traumatic scars is comprised of surgical and non-surgical interventions such as pressure therapy, silicone, corticosteroid, and radiotherapy... Recently, great progress in treating traumatic scars has been achieved by the development of novel technologies including laser, intense pulsed light (IPL), radiofrequency, and ultrasound" (2019). The article provides details on the effects of different lasers on scars. I encourage you to read it if you want to talk to your surgeon about using laser, IPL, radiofrequency or ultrasound on your scar: https://www.ncbi.nlm.nih.gov/pmc/articles/PMC6350396.

Platelet-Rich Plasma (PRP) and Scars

In the article "The evidence behind the use of platelet-rich plasma (PRP) in scar management: a literature review," published in Scars, Burns & Healing, Alser & Goutos say "Platelet-rich plasma (PRP) is an increasingly popular product used in a variety of medical, surgical and aesthetic interventions; it is derived by spinning down a patient's own blood and applying it back to an area of the body undergoing an intervention." The authors conducted a literature review and found "regarding surgical scars, the current data suggest that PRP may improve wound healing and early scar quality; furthermore, incorporation of PRP in fat-grafting procedures undertaken in conjunction with non-ablative, fractional laser can contribute to better wound healing as well as a significant improvement in texture, colour and contour in traumatic scar resurfacing" (Alser & Goutos, 2018).

Breast Surgery scars

Unsightly breast reduction scars may be complicated to treat. Engler says "scar revisions... are procedures, designed to improve the appearance of scars, in which the undesirable scars are removed and the skin is resewn with several layers of sutures under minimal or no tension. Steroids are often injected during and after this procedure to help prevent the scars from reforming" (2000).

Ask your surgeon when it is okay to begin using scar

massage techniques and other interventions like lasers and massage cupping on your breast scars.

Facial Surgery Scars

Many of my facelift clients are worried about the scar behind their ears. In their book *The Facelift Bible: Including the Facelift Diaries*, Sasada and Guest say "lumpiness of the scar does sometimes occur. This is usually minimal and primarily affects the skin behind the ear. It is due to the fact that the skin behind the ear is much thicker than elsewhere on the face. This may respond to massage and 'tincture of time'" (2016). Additionally, Perry says after a facelift, "small lumps are common and require massage" (2007). I will often feel harder sections of swelling in the face, particularly near the angle of the jaw and under the chin. These go away with continued manual lymphatic drainage massage and gentle lymphatic cupping. I have also felt interior stitches in the face and neck near the ear. These are usually dissolvable. Tell your surgeon if one of your stitches makes you feel nervous.

Abdominoplasty Scars

It's important to take good care of a tummy-tuck scar. The good news is that the angry red color does fade with time. It's important not to stretch or move around more than your surgeon allows. Engler explains that "in order to achieve the maximum cosmetic result, the abdominal tissues must be closed under a certain amount of tension; otherwise, the skin may be too loose, which partially defeats the purpose of the procedure. Excess tension increases the possibility of a less desirable scar" (2000). I'll have more advice for taking care of your tummy-tuck scar later in the chapter.

Is your tummy-tuck scar asymmetrical? In the article "Scar Asymmetry after Abdominoplasty: The Unexpected Role of Seroma" published in the *Annals of Plastic Surgery*, di Summa et al. say "silent seromas should be considered as a possible etiologic factor of scar asymmetries appearing during late follow-up after abdominoplasty." In some patients, "fibrous capsule due to chronic seromas resulted in abdominal scar deviation and asymmetry. Surgical capsulectomy followed by wearing of compressive garments resulted to be an effective treatment with pleasant aesthetic outcome and no seroma recurrence" (2013). Ask your physician to perform ultrasonography if you suspect you have an encapsulated chronic seroma.

Liposuction Scars

The American Society for Aesthetic Plastic Surgery (ASAPS) says "there are two types of marks that can remain on the skin after liposuction. One is a true scar and the other is known as dyschromia, which is a dark (hyperpigmented) or light (hypopigmented) spot on the skin" (Liposuction, 2018). Some of my clients have sunken liposuction cannula scars, especially on their torso. Engler says irregularities in liposuction scars "may be due to the trauma of the back and forth motion of the cannula as it passes repeatedly through the incision in the skin, to a slight over-resection (removal) of fat in that region since more cannula strokes occur there, or both" (2000).

Open or Closed Liposuction Incisions

Leaving liposuction incisions open allows fluid to drain from the body, but it can be messy for the patient to care for their constantly draining wounds. Engler usually does not leave his incisions open because "an incision that has been sutured will normally produce a better (less noticeable) scar than one that has been left open" (2000).

How To Take Care of Your Scar

First things first—Treat your scars gently! Please do not dry brush or try to exfoliate your surgical scar.

I found that using a silicone scar sheet did help my facial surgery scar. In the article "Overview of Surgical Scar Prevention and Management" published in the *Journal of Korean Medical Science*, Son & Harjian say "silicone gel sheets or silicone oil-based cream has been proved to be effective in limiting hypertrophic growth of scars." Using silicone increases skin hydration and temperature. The authors recommend that people at risk for developing hypertrophic scars start using silicone gel sheets "as early as two weeks after an operation ... every two hours with 30-[minute] rest intervals between. The interval is gradually increased to four hours with 30-[minute] rest intervals. This is continued for up to six months after the operation" (2014). Fu et al. explain that "silicone products (silicone gel, sheet, strip, cream, spray, or foam) are thought to be capable to effectively inhibit the hyperplasia of scar by multiple mechanisms including hydration, polarization of scar tissue, and elevation of local oxygen tension" (2019).

Ask your surgeon if it is okay to use silicone or any of the following methods to help heal your scar before trying them yourself. It is usually recommended that clients wait several weeks before using silicone scar products.

What about natural treatments our parents or grandparents might recommend? In the article "Nutritional Support for Wound Healing," MacKay and Miller say "post-operative topical application of Aloe vera and Centella asiatica extracts may facilitate the creation of a flexible, fine scar with high tensile strength at the wound site" (2003). Additionally, Bylka et al. say in the article, "Centella Asiatica in Cosmetology," published in *Advances in Dermatology and Allergology/Postępy Dermatologii i Alergologii,* "Centella asiatica* (Gotu kola) is effective in treatment of wounds, also in infective wounds, burns, and hypertrophic scar" and that "the mechanism of action involves promoting fibroblast proliferation and increasing the synthesis of collagen and intracellular fibronectin content and also improvement of the tensile strength of newly formed skin as well as inhibiting the inflammatory phase of hypertrophic scars and keloids" (2013).

In the article "Inhibitory Activities of Omega-3 Fatty Acids and Traditional African Remedies on Keloid Fibroblasts," Olaitan et al. say "shea butter is traditionally used as a skin care product due to its hydrating properties and its ability to soften scar tissues" and "oils rich in omega-3 fatty acids may be effective in reducing actively proliferating keloid fibroblasts" (2011). Make sure shea butter is completely absorbed by your skin before you put on your compression garment and be sure to check with your surgeon before trying any of these treatments.

Does the Orientation of a Scar Matter?

Langer lines follow the natural orientation of collagen fibers in the skin. If an incision doesn't follow these lines, it may affect how nicely the scar heals. Skin tape is a great tool to reduce tension on new scars. (Don't confuse it with kinesiotaping!) In the article "A Randomized, Controlled Trial to Determine the Efficacy of Paper Tape in Preventing Hypertrophic Scar Formation in Surgical Incisions that Traverse Langer's Skin Tension Line," Atkinson et al. say "paper tape is likely to be an effective modality for the prevention of hypertrophic scarring through its ability to eliminate scar tension" (Atkinson et al, 2005). If you have developed hypertrophic or keloid scars in the past, ask your plastic surgeon if using skin tape is right for you.

Helping Older Scars

How can you help your scars? Massage! In the article "Up-to-date Approach to Manage Keloids and Hypertrophic Scars: a Useful Guide," published in *Burns: Journal of the International Society for Burn Injuries*, Arno et al. say "massage therapy, manual or mechanical ... is standard therapy in rehabilitation centers specializing in the treatment of scars and burns. Although there is no scientific evidence, it has been shown that massage therapy not only reduces scar-related pain and itching, but also increases range of motion" (2014).

If you have reduced range of motion or increased sensitivity around your surgery scars, incorporating five to ten minutes of scar massage into your regular hour-long massage sessions can bring relief. Scar massage techniques can be used by a specially trained massage therapist, occupational therapist or physical therapist, with your surgeon's permission, starting two months after your surgery. I have advanced training in post-oncologic breast surgery scar massage and have also worked with plastic, orthopedic and cardiothoracic surgery scars.

Once you have your doctor's permission to start massaging your surgery area, here are my tips for self-massage on scars:

* Let scars heal for at least two months before starting self-massage

- Use a small amount of oil (spot test to make sure you are not allergic)
- Use light pressure, move slowly, and stop if skin becomes red or little red dots form on the skin
- Use special scar massage strokes (watch massage therapist Heather Wibbels' video at https://youtu.be/1vMvAJYikxo)
- Focus on moving the scar and skin horizontally instead of pushing down
- Limit self-massage on scars to less than five minutes a day

Dermarolling for scars and stretch marks?

The RealSelf website is a great resource to research questions relating to plastic surgery recovery. Clients ask the questions and plastic surgeons from across the country answer them. One method I have heard of recently is using a dermarolling device to remodel older scar tissue. See answers to the question "Is it true that dermaroller can treat old scars and stretch marks?" at https://www.realself.com/question/philippines-ph-true-dermaroller-treat-scars-and-stretch-marks#1570468.

Find more tips at RealSelf.com and create a profile so you can start asking questions. My profile is at https://www.realself.com/user/3190163.

The Future: No Scars at All?

Did you know that when fetal surgery is performed in the womb, the baby is born without any scars? George F. Murphy, MD, a Professor of Pathology at Harvard Medical School and co-lead of the HSCI Skin Program, is focusing on using skin stem cells to heal wounds "by regenerating tissue instead of forming a scar," which is what happens when we are injured before we are born (Healing Without Scars, 2018). Hopefully this research will find a way to use stem cells to completely eliminate the body's need to form a scar after an injury.

What are some ways you have healed your scars in the past? Did your parents or grandparents have a home remedy that worked? Write that advice here:

_____

_____

What are those lumps and bumps after liposuction?

Most if not all of my liposuction clients start to feel lumps a few months after their surgery. Schafer says "lumps can be caused by scar tissue forming unevenly. Massaging the area helps smooth these imperfections." Schafer also says "contour irregularities include dimpling, rippling, bagginess and lumps. Most of these issues are improved with massage, ... external ultrasound and exercise to help increase blood circulation" (2001).

Why Am I Lumpy After Liposuction?

Dixit and Wagh (2013) outline four reasons for lumps and bumps after liposuction:

- liposuction too close to the surface of the skin
- fibrotic adhesions
- loose skin
- not wearing your compression garment properly

How can we tell these reasons apart?

Dixit and Wagh say "surface dents due to excessive superficial liposuction persist on skin retraction and in the supine position. Dents due to fibrous adhesions to underlying muscle worsen on muscle contraction and dents due to skin redundancy may improve on supine position, but will definitely improve on skin retraction" (2013). McNemar et al. say treatment of the inner thighs often brings less even results than the outer thigh because "the thin, delicate skin on the inner thighs is more likely to reveal any irregularities or unevenness under the skin" (2006).

Treatment for loose skin

How long will loose skin last after liposuction surgery? Engler says "the absorption of swelling and the redraping of the skin can take several weeks or months" (2000). Dixit and Wagh recommend that "patients with the possibility of residual skin laxity must also be informed that they would need to wear the compression garment for a longer period, beyond the usual 6 weeks up to 8–12 weeks to encourage/allow the maximum possible skin retraction to take place" (2013). If loose skin persists for more than six months, talk to your plastic surgeon about skin tightening options.

Treatment for Lumps, Bumps and Fibrosis

First, what is fibrosis? We have all felt it — the lumps, bumps and firm spots under the skin in the months and years after surgery. In the article "Cellular and Molecular Mechanisms of Fibrosis," published in the *Journal of Pathology*, Wynn says "fibrosis is defined by the overgrowth, hardening, and/or scarring of various tissues and is attributed to excess deposition of extracellular matrix components including collagen. Fibrosis is the end result of chronic inflammatory reactions induced by a variety of stimuli including persistent infections, autoimmune reactions, allergic responses, chemical insults, radiation, and tissue injury" (2008).

In the Liposuction Complications chapter of the book *Safe Liposuction and Fat Transfer*, Tremblay et al. say "liposuction near the subcutaneous-dermal plane is believed to stimulate collagen formation which usually results in a desirable retraction of redundant skin.

Some patients may develop an exaggerated fibroblastic response resulting in significant subcutaneous induration" (Narins, 2003, 344).

In the article "Effect of Abdominal Liposuction on Sonographically Guided High—Intensity Focused Ultrasound Ablation," published in the *Journal of Ultrasound Medicine*, Zhao et al. say liposuction can cause fibrosis because it "alters the tissue structure of the abdominal wall" and "these alterations result in subcutaneous tissue fibrosis and scar formation, which may explain why the abdominal walls of the patients who had liposuction did not feel rubbery" (2014).

Wynn mentions that fibrosis is linked to inflammation. In the article "The Inflammation–fibrosis Link? A Jekyll and Hyde Role for Blood Cells During Wound Repair," published in the Journal of Investigative Dermatology, Stramer et al. found that "adult tissue repair always leads to formation of a fibrotic scar where the wound has healed. In recent years, it has become clear that the wound inflammatory response may be, at least in part, responsible for fibrosis at sites of tissue repair." Is the key to just stop inflammation? Not so fast! Stramer et al. also found that "there is still much evidence that inflammation has an important part to play in orchestrating adult tissue repair and that a gross blockade of the inflammatory response, even in the presence of the best antibiotics, would not be a useful clinical therapy" (2007).

How does fibrosis differ from the thick, hard swelling present in the first weeks after surgery? Wynn says "in contrast to acute inflammatory reactions, which are characterized by rapidly resolving vascular changes, oedema and neutrophilic inflammation, fibrosis typically results from chronic inflammation—defined as an immune response that persists for several months and in which inflammation, tissue remodelling and repair processes occur simultaneously" and that "fibrosis occurs when the synthesis of new collagen by myofibroblasts exceeds the rate at which it is degraded, such that the total amount of collagen increases over time" (2008).

If you perform an Internet search for fibrosis, you'll learn that fibrosis can happen in organs, too. Stramer at al. say "fibrosis is certainly not unique to repair of skin tissues. Every organ of the body can mount a repair response that generally results in a fibrotic lesion" (2017).

So fibrosis is due to chronic inflammation and is the hardening and scarring of tissues. I owe a huge debt to Certified Lymphedema Therapist Karen Ashforth for sharing her insights in understanding and treating fibrosis in clients with lymphedema—it has improved my treatment of post-surgical clients. Ashforth says there are two different types of fibrosis: soft and woody. Soft fibrosis is created by lymphatic stasis. Hard fibrosis is scar tissue from surgery, radiation or cellulitis. Additionally, the tissue can have one of two presentations: either a gel or a woody texture.

Ashforth encourages Certified Lymphedema Therapists to track their progress by rating the tissue extensibility before and after each treatment—how much farther does the skin and underlying tissue move in every direction after a massage session? Knowing this will enable you to track how well manual lymphatic drainage and other massage techniques are working to help you heal after surgery.

How can we help reduce those lumps and bumps? First let's look at boards and foam pieces.

Abdominal and Lumbar Boards

Some plastic surgeons recommend that their liposuction clients use abdominal boards and others do not recognize their effectiveness. Many abdominal liposuction clients use abdominal boards because they help support good posture which reduces skin irregularities during the healing process. M&D is one popular brand.

Sotelo-Paz recommends her liposuction clients wear abdominal and lumbar boards. She recommends that abdominal boards be worn starting the day after liposuction surgery, but only during the day. Sotelo-Paz tell her clients to wear an abdominal board under their compression garment and over a thin tank top and sheet of lipo foam. She recommends that clients "place the lumbar board under your lipo foams and the tip of the lumbar board should go right above your butt crack. You should start wearing this one day after surgery and keep wearing it for one month" (2016).

Abdominal boards may not be indicated for tummy tuck clients; make sure you have permission from your surgeon before you use an abdominal board after abdominoplasty or liposuction.

For clients with lymphedema, we recommend using a base layer next to the skin (usually stockinette), then a layer of foam that wraps all the way around the limb, then layers of short stretch compression bandages. This layering "recipe" can be adapted for post-surgical use by replacing the stockinette with a thin tank top or micromassage garment.

If you feel hot or sweaty in your compression, try using a tank top made of bamboo or a wicking garment.

Compression bandaging used for reducing edema in a person with lymphedema includes several layers of material, including a stretchable layer for protecting the skin and absorbing perspiration, a layer of smooth or uneven padding, often made of foam, and the bandage-style compression itself (Foldi & Foldi, 2012, 529–532). For post-surgical swelling, a tank top can be used as the bottom later and foam pieces for the padding.

One way to layer your compression:

- Abdomen compression layers: tank top, foam, abdominal board, compression garment
- Flank compression layers: tank top, foam, compression garment
- Back compression layers: tank top, lumbar board, foam, compression garment

Foam Padding to Reduce Fibrosis

As I mentioned earlier, I first learned about the use of foam as a treatment for clients with advanced lymphedema. Different types of foam can be used for controlling both swelling and fibrosis. An insert made of chip foam or a foam piece designed with channels or dots may be a good option if fibrotic tissue has formed on the limbs or torso. Many lymphedema clinics use similar techniques to reduce fibrosis in their patients. For example, Ashforth shares that the Dominican Santa Cruz Hospital's clinic uses "chip foam and cherry pit compression pads and garments, textured elastic compression garments, specialised manual techniques, such as myofascial release and instrument-aided soft tissue mobilisation, and pneumatic compression to ameliorate brawny hard swelling that does not recede with elevation" (2011).

In the book *Compression Bandaging for Lymphedema Management*, Klose says "softening and breaking up of this fibrotic tissue is obtained by including foam rubber padding materials (e.g. **Komprex®**) within a moderately tight bandage. This achieves a localized pressure increase in this area. Muscular activity further acts upon these fibrotic areas, loosening and breaking up the accumulated deposits of scar and connective tissue" (2010). Yes, you should exercise with your foam sheets. Movement will encourage the loosening and breaking up of fibrosis that Klose mentions.

Some surgeons give their patients surgical foam, and sometimes it is attached to the body for the first few days after surgery. These foam pieces should not be completely soaked with water. To dry this type of foam, towel dry first and then use a hairdryer on a cool air setting.

I also use foam chips, shapes or sheets of channel or polka dot foam placed underneath your compression garment to break down fibrosis by subtly kneading the hardened areas as you move throughout the day. Chip bags are named "Schneider packs," after their inventor, Bernd Schneider, a Senior Therapist at the Foeldi Clinic in Hinterzarten, Germany. If you would like extra sheets, they are called **Medi® Lymphpads®**. **Komprex®** foam rubber shapes are "used to amplify compression, soften fibrosis, as well as to provide padding" (Komprex, n.d.).

The channel and polka dot foam sheets I stock in my office are machine-washable and dryer-friendly. Joint movement exercises performed while wearing foam sheets and your compression garment will work gently to break up fibrosis over time. Some of my clients will use their first, slightly larger compression garment when exercising, shower and then change into their smaller garment. Be sure your skin has completely absorbed any lotion or oil before you use these foam sheets.

Ashforth created the cherry pit pack, another option for breaking down fibrotic tissue. A study by Ashforth et al. titled "A New Treatment for Soft Tissue Fibrosis in the Breast" published in the *Journal of Lymphoedema*, found that women with swelling and fibrotic tissue who received lymphatic drainage massage and wore a **JoViPitPak®** under their elastic compression garment for two hours each day for three weeks had "decreased tissue density" and, "increased perceived cosmesis" (cosmetic appearance) (2011). Cherry pit packs can also be tucked inside a pneumatic compression massage device to reduce fibrosis and mimic the massaging effect of exercise with compression.

Pitpaks® may look small, but they are very aggressive form of treatment. Please use them cautiously. Ashforth recommends that clients start by just using them for 30 minutes and build up time, monitoring skin for tolerance. They should not be used on fragile skin or areas with poor sensation. Learn more about **JoViPitPaks®** here: https://youtu.be/kknHwhEGuLg.

During Your Massage Session

The first few visits after a liposuction surgery are focused on reducing swelling. When I start to feel fibrosis, lumps or bumps forming under your skin (usually a few months after surgery), I will use one or more methods to help break it up and help give you the results you want from your liposuction. Here are a few of the tricks up my sleeve:

Deeper Massage Techniques

Many clients mention that their torso feels stuck and glued down first thing in the morning. Stretching their torso feels like pulling taffy. I start with hands-on targeted deep techniques including pin-and-stretch and myofascial scar work to break up your lumps and bumps, increase your range of motion and give you a more open feeling. Adding hot stones to the massage warms the tissues and allows me to work deeper without the client feeling pain. The key to fibrosis massage is a sustained compression of the tissue over time. The therapist may use a pair of medical gloves or a piece of **Dycem®**, a special polymer with very high grip properties, to increase the effectiveness of the massage.

Soft Tissue Mobilization: IASTM or ASTYM

Instrument Assisted Soft Tissue Mobilization is used to treat fascia restrictions and soft tissue fibrosis. An article titled "Instrument Assisted Soft Tissue Mobilisation (IASTM)" by the Ohio Valley Medical Center says "microtrauma initiates reabsorption of inappropriate fibrosis or excessive scar tissue and facilitates a cascade of healing activities resulting in remodeling of affected soft tissue structures. Adhesions within the soft tissue which may have developed as a result of surgery, immobilization, repeated strain or other mechanisms, are broken down allowing full functional restoration to occur" (2019). IASTM shouldn't hurt or leave a bruise.

In the article "**Astym**® Therapy: a Systematic Review," published in the *Annals of Translational Medicine*, Chughtai et al. say **Astym**® "was developed to address soft-tissue dysfunctions by stimulating the regeneration of soft tissues and the resorption of inappropriate scar tissue/ fibrosis." How does it work? The technique encourages the body to use "cellular mediators and growth factors to assist in activating scar tissue resorption, stimulating tissue turnover and regenerating soft tissues" (2019).

It is important NOT to take an NSAID medication if we do deeper soft tissue mobilization work in your massage session. Allowing inflammation to occur is an essential part of the healing process. I mention more about NSAID medications in the Wound Healing chapter.

Lymphatic Massage Cupping
(Myofascial Decompression)

Massage Cupping is one type of myofascial decompression. There are several different types of cupping, and I specifically use a type that is gentler and more dynamic than traditional cupping. There is no pain, no bruising and no red circles after this lymphatic-focused cupping! Massage Cupping uses suction to create negative pressure in the tissues of the body. Massage Cupping after surgery should be done with an awareness of the lymphatic system, since the fluids brought up near the skin's surface are removed from the body by the lymphatic system.

One brand is **LymphaTouch®**. In the article "Negative pressure therapy in the management of lymphoedema," published in the *Journal of Lymphoedema*, Gott et al. say that negative pressure massage therapy devices like the **LymphaTouch®** can be "targeted directly over scars, areas of radiation induced fibrosis, fibrosis from lymphoedema" (2018).

In my office, I use a cupping machine that provides either a steady or pulsating level of suction. Silicone cups can be used at home if a manual treatment is desired. Oil is applied to the skin (I use jojoba oil or arnica oil) and the cups are used at the gentlest level of pressure. I manually treat the lymph nodes in the neck, abdomen and inguinal areas (also axillae lymph nodes if the upper body is being treated) using manual lymphatic drainage techniques, so the lymph nodes are primed to accept and filter the swelling. I love using lymphatic-focused massage cupping on my clients and have found it is gentle enough to help even those over 70 years of age who have had liposuction.

How To Prepare For a Fibrosis Massage Session

I use either heat or cooling techniques to help my clients get the most from a fibrosis massage session.

If I opt to use heat, I will turn to my hot stones! Most clients find adding hot stones to their session makes them much more relaxed. I find that they allow me to do deeper work without causing discomfort to my clients.

Cooling is also an option. In a study titled "Local Skin Cooling as an Aid to the Management of Patients with Breast Cancer Related Lymphedema and Fibrosis of the Arm or Breast," published in *Lymphology*, Mayrovitz, Harvey, & Yzer found that using two to four washcloths cooled in an ice water bath and applied to cool fibrotic tissue for twelve to fifteen minutes before a manual lymphatic drainage session helped with fibrosis. The study found that after the cooling washcloth treatment, "myofascial lengthening, scar tissue releasing, and other aspects of treatment are easier to perform thereby reducing treatment time and effort while achieving improved functional mobility" (2017).

Other Modalities for Fibrosis

A small study published in the *Annals of Rehabilitation Medicine* titled "Clinical Outcomes of Extracorporeal Shock Wave Therapy in Patients With Secondary Lymphedema: A Pilot Study," by Bae & Kim found that Extracorporeal Shockwave Therapy (ESWT) had an effect on fibrosis in patients with lymphedema (Bae & Kim, 2013).

According to the article "Cellulite and Focused Extracorporeal Shockwave Therapy for Non-invasive Body Contouring: a Randomized Trial," published in *Dermatology and Therapy*, ESWT may also reduce cellulite, including dimples in the gluteal area (Knobloch et al, 2013). How does it work? ESWT uses the same technology that is used to break up kidney stones.

In the article "**Role of HIVAMAT** ® 200 (deep oscillation) in the treatment of the lymphedema of the limbs," published in the *European Journal of Lymphology and Related Problems*, Gasbarro et al. found that deep oscillation aided massage helped reduce fibrosis. The Hivamat product uses intermittent electrostatic fields with deep oscillation and has also been found to reduce edema (Gasbarro, 2006).

Help Yourself at Home

Once your surgeon clears you for vigorous exercise, consider using at-home techniques to reduce scar tissue and fibrosis.

Self-massage tools like the **Coregeous**® ball, an air-filled sponge ball, may help. According to Jill Miller, the inventor of the **Coregeous**® ball, "the balls' grippiness maximizes their ability to create shear, and their pliable density allows them to conform without injuring the tissues on knobby bony prominences." Miller's book The Roll Model provides a step-by-step sequence for pin/spin and mobilize and other shear techniques for the torso ons pages 170–184 and routines that can be used on the arms and legs are featured later in the book. I also urge you to read the story of a woman who uses the ball to reduce her chronic scar tissue discomfort after two cesarean sections and a liver operation (she donated part of her liver to a colleague who needed a transplant) (2014).

To get an idea of what the treatment looks like, view these videos:

"How To Get Rid of Abdominal Scar Tissue with Jill Miller": https://youtu.be/Px7AqK2bBsg

Techniques for the flanks: https://youtu.be/BxrWy23m_48

Inner thigh fibrosis in "Therapy balls for knees: adductors": https://youtu.be/gXAU7QRUyUE

Another at-home option is to use a block to change scar tissue. Certified Athletic Therapist Deanna Hansen is the creator of Block Therapy. She had a breast reduction in her twenties and found that "over the years, the scar tissue began to adhere to my ribcage." According to the

Block Therapy website, the practice involves lying "on a therapeutic tool called the Block Buddy for a minimum of three minutes in various positions throughout the body." (n.d.)

Also consider working with fibrosis using exercise by trying a slow, stretching yoga practice. They key is to hold the poses for several breaths. One example, taught by yoga instructor and author Candace Moore, is at https://youtu.be/SAcU0E6mOQw.

What's With All The "Homework?"

Silicone cups, exercises, abdominal boards, foam pieces, self-massage, balls and blocks. Why do I give my clients so much "homework" after surgery to reduce swelling and fibrosis? Let me explain it using NEAT, a concept I first learned from exercise physiologist Fabio Comana when studying for my Certificate in Fitness Instruction/Exercise Science at UCSD Extension.

According to Dr. James Levine from the Endocrine Research Unit at the Mayo Clinic, non-exercise activity thermogenesis (NEAT) is "the energy expended for everything we do that is not sleeping, eating or sports-like exercise" (2004). The positive effects of all the non-exercise low intensity activities that we do each day can really add up and have a larger effect than just relying on three or four formal bouts of exercise.

It's the same way with healing from plastic surgery—the little things we do all day add up. I believe it's as important for my clients to actively participate in their own healing as it is to come to their manual lymphatic drainage appointments.

"Style is knowing who you are, what you want to say, and not giving a damn." — Gore Vidal

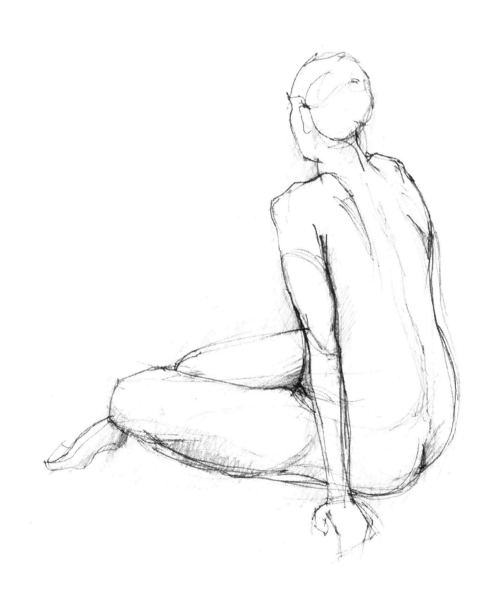

CHAPTER 6
WOUND HEALING

The Itching!

It is completely normal to feel itchy. How can we treat itchiness after surgery? In the article, "Postburn Itch: A Review of the Literature," published in Wounds : a compendium of clinical research and practice, Nedelec & Lasalle state that "the environmental and physical factors that increase itch are dryness, hot environments or warm water, physical effort, sweating and fatigue." They mentioned several types of nonpharmacological interventions, including "moisturizers, cooling, TENS, massage, pressure garments, low-level laser" (Nedelec & Lasalle, 2018). TENS is short for Transcutaneous Electrical Nerve Stimulation. Garments can make skin drier than usual, so be sure to remember to moisturize regularly.

One natural remedy for itching is oatmeal. In the article "Oatmeal in dermatology: A brief review," published in the Indian Journal of Dermatology, Venereology and Leprology, Pazyar et al. state that "oatmeal has been used for centuries to decrease itching in a variety of xerotic dermatoses" because it "possesses different types of phenols which exert the antioxidant and anti-inflammatory activity" (Pazyar et al., 2012). An easy way to take advantage of the benefits of oatmeal is to use a soap, body wash or lotion that contains collodial oatmeal.

How to Heal Faster

Unlike a tumble on the playground, healing after plastic surgery takes more than a kiss and a bandage. There are some simple tips you can follow that will allow your body to heal itself faster.

My first three wound healing tips focus on keeping warm, drinking water and controlling your pain levels. In the article "Preventing and Managing Surgical Wound Dehiscence," published in Advances in Skin and Wound Care, Doughty says "wound healing requires oxygen and nutrients, and that delivery of these key ingredients to the wound site depends on adequate perfusion, control of edema, adequate nutrient intake, and normal oxygenation." Doughty recommends that "during the early postoperative period, healing strategies include: maintaining blood volume through adequate fluid replacement, maintaining warmth (to prevent vasoconstriction), aggressively managing pain (to prevent vasoconstriction)" (2005).

Don't Smoke

It is extremely important NOT to smoke before and after surgery. According to Sasada and Guest, "smoking is associated with at least a ten-fold incidence of wound infection and skin necrosis" (2016). Anderson and Hamm explain why, stating "tobacco altogether slows collagen production, weakens scar tissue, and leaves healed tissues more susceptible to risk of recurrent injury. These effects can alter all phases of wound healing, thereby resulting in inefficient and slower closure of wounds" (2014). And yes, those new popular e-cigarettes are also detrimental for wound healing (Smith, 2017).

Quit and Stay Quit Monday is a free online program that can help you quit smoking. Visit the website at https://www.iquitmonday.org.

Don't Get Drunk

It's also important not to drink alcohol to excess while you are healing from surgery. A study in mice performed at the Burn and Shock Trauma Institute, Loyola University Medical Center, found that "a single ethanol exposure equivalent to moderate intoxication (100 mg/dl) can dramatically impair the proliferative phase of dermal wound healing" (Radek et al., 2005). McNemar et al. recommend that their patients "don't drink any alcohol for about ten days because it can dilate the blood vessels and increase postoperative bleeding" (2006).

Eat Healthy

This advice is especially important if you have temporary weight loss or gastric bypass surgery. Olesen & Olesen say "following gastric bypass surgery (and even after weight loss from dieting), calcium, vitamin B12, and iron levels tend to be low. Most patients are advised to take multivitamins, B12, calcium, and iron for a year or longer after completion of their surgery" (2005).

Vitamin C is also important! In the article "Vitamin C and Immune Function," published in Nutrients, Carr & Maggini say "Vitamin C deficiency is the fourth leading nutrient deficiency in the United States." Why is taking vitamin C especially important after surgery? Because "vitamin C deficiency results in impaired immunity and higher susceptibility to infections. In turn, infections significantly impact on vitamin C levels due to enhanced inflammation and metabolic requirement." (2017). Ask your doctor when it's okay to start consuming Vitamin C after surgery.

In the article "Nutritional Support for Wound Healing," MacKay and Miller (2003) say "nutritional deficiencies can impede wound healing, and several nutritional factors required for wound repair may improve healing time and wound outcome" and share information about how nutrition can help heal the body naturally, I highly recommend reading this article. Find it online at http://archive. foundationalmedicinereview.com/component/docman/ doc_download/286-review-article-nutritional-support-for-wound-healing?Itemid=485 (must be registered at foundationalmedicinereview.com to download).

Be Cautious About Supplements

Should you take supplements for healing? Social media ads and alternative medicine websites can convince us we will never be truly healthy unless we swallow a handful of pills every day. Your surgeon's advice may be different. Engler recommends that "in general, for a period of three weeks before and after surgery, all nonessential medications and preparations should be discontinued" (2000). Sasada and Guest share that "we advise our patients to stop taking all herbal medicines, vitamins and food supplements two weeks before surgery and to resume two weeks after surgery" (2016).

Shiffman recommends that liposuction patients "not take any vitamins, especially vitamins C and E for 2 weeks prior to surgery AND for 1 week after surgery. Discontinue all hormones (check with your physician first) 3 weeks prior to surgery and for 2 weeks after surgery. Try not to schedule surgery on a day close to your menstrual period. It is preferable not to do surgery the first 5 days of menstrual bleeding" (2006, 97).

Don't Overtreat Your Pain

Be careful with taking NSAIDS. Anderson and Hamm say "non-steroidal anti-inflammatory drugs (NSAIDs) have been shown to have a depressant effect on wound healing while simultaneously decreasing the granulocytic inflammatory reaction. NSAIDs inhibit the production of

PGE2, an inflammatory mediating prostaglandin, and can thereby reduce pain. The suppression of PGE2 also occurs with excessive wound scarring and therefore NSAIDs may increase scar formation, especially if they are used during the proliferative phase of healing. NSAIDs have an anti-proliferative effect on blood vessels and skin, thereby delaying healing rate" (2014). Fu et al. share that "inflammation is crucial to the removal of dead tissue and the prevention of infection by neutrophils and macrophages through the actions of phagocytosis and the secretion of proteases and cytokines. A moderate amount of inflammation is vital to the wound healing process for transition from the inflammatory phase to the proliferative phase" (2019). Acetaminophen is a non-NSAID pain reliever.

DO Treat Your Stress

What do you hear from your plastic surgeon? Take it easy. Take it easy. Take it easy. That's because reducing stress is important for your healing. In her book *108 Pearls to Awaken Your Healing Potential*, integrative cardiologist Dr. Mimi Guarneri says "stress is our immune system's nemesis. Not only do we get sick more easily under stress, we find it more difficult to recover" (2017).

The DeStress Monday website shares regular tips and guides to help you start every week with a positive frame of mind. Visit the website at https://www.destressmonday.org.

In the article "The Impact of Psychological Stress on Wound Healing: Methods and Mechanisms' published in Critical Care Nursing Clinics of North America, Gouin et al. say "psychological distress thus appears to influence recovery from medical procedures and healing of chronic wounds in clinical settings." To reduce stress, try journaling, aerobic exercise (with your surgeon's permission) and enjoying positive interactions with friends and loved ones (2012).

Speaking of positive interactions, your spouse can help with wound healing! According to an article titled "Hostile Marital Interactions, Proinflammatory Cytokine Production, and Wound Healing" published in the Archives of General Psychiatry, patients who discussed a marital disagreement for thirty minutes with a spouse experienced slower wound healing (Kiecolt-Glaser et al., 2005). Keep interactions positive!

Protect Your Incisions

If you are worried about putting pressure on your breasts or abdomen after a breast augmentation or tummy tuck, there are padded seat belt covers available to reduce the pressure caused by a seat belt.

Protect Any Transferred Fat

I do not perform manual lymphatic drainage massage or

any type of massage over or near areas with a fat transfer for at least a few weeks after surgery.

There is no research to back this, but many doctors and patients strongly recommend using an off-loading pillow, often called a BBL pillow, to take pressure off your bottom while sitting after fat grafting for gluteal augmentation (often called Brazilian Butt Lift, or BBL surgery). There are a few different pillows on the market, so find the one that is right for you. Proper posture and the ability to sit comfortably for longer periods of time are two important considerations.

If you have had a fat transfer to your outer thigh or gluteal area, choose a compression garment that does not compress the area. One option for post BBL and fat transfer to the thighs is the St. Azar Traditional Faja custom garment from Curvy Gyals.

Complications

Faja Burn

Faja burn is a term that people who have had surgery use to describe a wide variety of tissue breakdown after surgery, from abrasions to more serious cases of eschar (see "When is a Scab Not a Scab?" below) or necrosis. Skin abrasions can be a signal that your compression garment is too tight or doesn't fit properly. Compression garments should feel snug but not uncomfortable. I have seen an abrasion-type faja burn on a client shortly after they sized down into a too-tight compression garment a few months after surgery.

Sometimes an improperly fitting compression garment can do more harm than good. What can you do if you experience a skin abrasion from friction or excessive compression caused by your garment? Wearing a properly fitting compression garment and covering the abraded area with a piece of Sigvaris BiaSoft Fleece Padding Bandage may resolve the issue. Contact your surgeon if it gets worse or doesn't start to heal.

Wearing the garment can dry out your skin so keep yourself well moisturized.

Faja burns can also happen if skin folds are pushed together in a compression garment, especially if there is no tank top or foam between the skin and the compression garment.

Consult with your surgeon if your compression garment is irritating your skin.

When is a Scab Not a Scab?

According to Heather Flexer, DPT, CWS and owner and consultant at Better Wounds, "a scab is a collection of dried blood or drainage. Typically, brownish in color and limited to the incision line, suture or staple holes. Scabs will be easily removed after a shower and have healthy new pale pink skin underneath. Eschar is completely different. Eschar is dead devitalized tissue resulting from a lack of oxygen or blood flow. It is typically black, thick and there may be pus along the edges. Trying to remove eschar will reveal a deeper wound however leaving it present might cause further damage. Dead tissue requires debridement and you should contact your surgeon. Be advised that some surgeons will recommend you continue with covering your wound with gauze despite research to support use of more advanced products (Wodash, 2013). For instance, honey-based products (Schell et al., 2019) or enzymatic debriders like collagenase are more active in selectively debriding devitalized tissues and result in less painful dressing changes. If you experience a sudden increase in pain, drainage, odor from the area or general feelings of malaise; you should go to the Emergency Department as you may have an infection" (H. Flexer, personal communication, 2019).

Skin Necrosis

Necrosis means death of a cell; in this case, skin cells. It usually happens as a result of a limited oxygen and blood supply. In the article "Managing Complications in Abdominoplasty: A Literature Review" published in *Archives of Plastic Surgery*, Vidal et al. gave advice on dealing with necrosis, which may manifest with "signs of insufficient irrigation, such as delayed capillary fill and diminished local temperature." The healing process can take from weeks to months and treatment includes debridement and dressing of the wound as well as emotional support (2017). Dixit & Wagh recommend treatment including "surgical debridement, antibiotics and hyperbaric oxygen therapy." Remember that chronic smokers who have not stopped smoking are at high risk for skin necrosis (2013). If you suspect an infection, call your surgeon for advice.

Infections

Signs of infection include feeling feverish, tired or weak, drainage or a bad smell coming from your wound, or a painful, sore, hot, or red wound.

Cellulitis is a serious bacterial infection. Signs of cellulitis are: redness spreading over an area, hot skin, pain, and increased swelling. You may also feel tired and weak, like you are coming down with the flu. It is important to seek medical attention if you suspect you have cellulitis.

Where do infections come from? Vidal et al. found that "skin bacterial flora accounts for the majority of infections after abdominoplasties, especially *Staphylococcus epidermidis, Streptococcus pyogenes*, and *S. aureus*, requiring second-line antibiotic therapy when these species present methicillin resistance" (2017).

If you suspect an infection, call your surgeon for advice.

Seromas

Seromas are a possible complication of surgery. According to Engler, "a seroma can form if the fluid is inadequately drained and/or continues to accumulate after the drains are removed. When seromas do occur, they are treated initially with aspiration (using a fine needle to withdraw the fluid), reinsertion of one or more drains, or a combination. When identified and treated early, this complication is usually transient and produces only minimal disturbance" (2000).

Drains can help reduce seroma formation. According to an article by Janis et al. titled "Strategies for postoperative seroma prevention: a systematic review" and published in *Plastic and Reconstructive Surgery*, "effective strategies for seroma prevention included the use of closed-suction drains; keeping the drains until their output volume was minimal; [and] maintaining a high pressure gradient in the drain" (2016).

Tell your surgeon about any seromas as soon as possible.

Treatments

Low-level Laser Therapy / Red LED / Photobiomodulation

I first experienced low-level laser therapy in my esthetician's office. The "red light" was used after my facial. Can a laser really make a difference? In the article "Mechanisms and applications of the anti-inflammatory effects of photobiomodulation" published in AIMS Biophysics, Hamblin says "low-level level laser therapy is the use of red and near-infrared light to stimulate healing, relieve pain, and reduce inflammation" and offers a nice overview of why this technology works at https://www.ncbi.nlm.nih.gov/pmc/articles/PMC5523874 (2017).

This therapy isn't just for beauty. BreastCancer.org says "low-level laser therapy has been cleared by the US Food and Drug Administration for the treatment of lymphedema" and "the thinking is that the laser light increases the flow of lymph, reduces the amount of excess protein and tissue in the fluid, and reduces the ability of scar tissue to 'stick' to the underlying healthy tissue" (Laser Therapy for Lymphedema, 2012).

Can it help after surgery? In the article "Phototherapy with Light Emitting Diodes: Treating a Broad Range of Medical and Aesthetic Conditions in Dermatology," published in the *Journal of Clinical and Aesthetic Dermatology*, Ablon says laser emitting diodes (LED) "in contrast with thermal-based skin-tightening devices, such as radiofrequency and focused ultrasound, LEDs do not produce thermal injury." Ablon shares a study where male and female subjects "underwent combined blepharoplasty and Er:YAG/CO2 laser ablative resurfacing. Subsequently, one-half of each subject's face was randomly selected and treated with a 633nm (96J/cm2) red LED for 20 minutes immediately after surgery, 48 hours post-surgery, and twice more the following week. Resolution of erythema, edema, bruising, and days to healing was assessed.... The LED-treated side healed after a mean (SD) of 13.5 ... days versus 26.8 ... days for the untreated side" (2018).

Ablon cautions that "while home use devices have been available for several years, there are many differences between those devices and those specifically designed for use by physicians. The home use devices necessarily deliver significantly less power and typically do not have light panel arrays large enough to treat the entire face at once" but says " in some cases, home units may be used adjunctively with dermatologist-provided treatment to address specific areas of concern" (2018). If you do decide to buy a device for home use, do your research. Some devices advertise themselves as FDA-approved, but they are only FDA-approved for use as a heat lamp.

Hyperbaric Oxygen Therapy (HBOT)

Receiving Hyperbaric Oxygen Therapy (HBOT) may help speed wound healing after surgery. Vidal et al. say "not only does hyperbaric oxygenation increase oxygen availability to different territories by increasing the partial pressure of O2, it also stimulates neovascularization, collagen production, fibroblast proliferation, and mobilization of stem cells from the bone marrow to the injured site" (2017).

Manuka Honey

Sood et al. reviewed studies that tested the effectiveness of Manuka Honey because of its role as "an ancient remedy for the treatment of infected wounds … first recognized as a topical antibacterial agent in 1892." They found that "in laboratory studies, Manuka honey has been shown to provide antibacterial action against a broad spectrum of bacteria and fungi," and "honey dressings make the wounds sterile in less time, enhance healing, and have a better outcome in terms of hypertrophic scars and postburn contractures" (2014). Be sure to ask your plastic surgeon before trying this treatment.

A Few Tips on Caring for Your Drains

Many surgeons use drains to help reduce swelling after surgery. One of my favorite clients nicknamed hers "the grenade!"

The Ohio State University Wexner Medical Center shares one way to clean the skin around your wound drain tube. They recommend you "start at the center where the tube comes out of the skin. Use a circular motion to clean the skin around the tube. Slowly move out and away from the tube 3 to 4 inches. Do not clean back towards the tube" (Home Care for Your Wound Drain, n.d.).

How can you know if your drain area might be infected? Call your doctor if you have redness greater than the size of a dime, swelling, heat, or pus around your drain insertion site. Your doctor may want to know if you are also running a fever, so take your temperature if you notice any of the signs listed above. After your drain is removed, don't submerge that part of your body in a bath or swimming pool until your incision is completely closed (Caring for Your Jackson-Pratt Drain, 2019).

If the amount of drainage suddenly decreases, ask your doctor if you should clear/strip/milk your drains. The "Caring for Your Jackson-Pratt Drain" article has a step-by-step guide to how to milk your drains at https://www.mskcc.org/cancer-care/patient-education/caring-your-jackson-pratt-drain.

How can you make sure your drains are safe while you are recovering? I have seen clients safety-pin drains to their compression garment or wear them in a t-shirt pocket. I have also seen bathrobes with drain pockets. My favorite way to handle drains is to use an apron-like drain pouch. It looks like a restaurant employee's apron and has large pockets and a long tie in the back. The apron allows you to move the drains as one unit without a lot of fumbling.

If you're thinking of buying anything fancy to hold your drains, remember that you will be inside and relaxing most of the time you are using drains. Save your money for buying new clothes instead!

If your drains are leaking fluid at the point where they enter the body, try the **Cutimed® Sorbion®** Sachet S Drainage wound dressing. It features a slit design down the middle to fit around the exit point of a drainage tube.

A Few Tips on Open Liposuction Incision Sites

When should you be alarmed by the drainage from an open incision? Shiffman says "the patient or caretaker should call the doctor if there is bright red bleeding through the dressings, drainage of pus, increasing pain, or other unusual symptoms (shortness of breath, abdominal pain, chest pain, mental confusion, etc.). Some pink drainage, not bright red drainage, is to be expected and may be quite profuse the first night" (2006, 99).

One client who had open liposuction incisions covered them with gauze and a **3M® Tegaderm®** Transparent Film Dressing to keep her clothes dry and clean while she was out of the house. I have also seen clients attach menstrual or incontinence pads to the back of their abdominal boards to catch fluid drainage.

Should you use gauze? Sood et al. say "Although gauze

has proven useful in many situations, clinicians and hospital staff must be aware when use of this material is not optimal. Woven gauze requires force to remove, and it can potentially lead to wound trauma and/or mechanical debridement. Residue left behind from woven gauze may allow the body to respond with granuloma formation" and "impregnated gauze does not absorb exudates and therefore does not have a role in wounds with a heavy drainage" (2014).

What's better than gauze for absorbing fluid from an open incision? One option is the **HK**® Super Absorbent Pad. Watch a video of Jeffrey Klein MD, the inventor of Tumescent Lidocaine Local Anesthesia, describing the pad at https://youtu.be/47VGEs4w90M. Another option is an abdominal pad dressing like the **Medline**® ABD latex-free sterile abdominal extra-absorbent pad. Monitor the health of your skin when you use a bandage under your compression—for some, when the dressing expands, it puts additional unwanted pressure on the body.

A Few Tips on Healing from Abdominal Etching

Wearing compression garments is an especially important part of recovery after abdominal etching. In the article "Abdominal Etching: Surgical Technique and Outcomes," published in *Plastic and Reconstructive Surgery*, Husain et al. say "the abdominal binder with TopiFoam is worn for 2 to 3 days until initial drainage has stopped. After that point, a compression garment is worn at all times for 2 weeks and part-time (approximately 12 hours/day) for an additional 2 weeks." How do they use **TopiFoam®**? They explain that "the etched lines are maintained by placing compression over the etched areas. TopiFoam (Mentor-Aesthetics, Irvine, Calif.) is cut to size over the etched areas into thin strips 1 cm in width to ensure the skin sticks down to the abdominal wall. Larger pieces of TopiFoam are placed on top of the existing ones for more uniform compression. An abdominal binder is used to secure the TopiFoam compression" (2019).

It is important to prevent seromas after this surgery. Husain et al. share that "the prevention of seroma complication is a key technical issue" and "the compression garment is extremely important in the abdominal etching patient, as even minor seromas can have a disastrous consequence with regard to the desired results" (2019).

A Few Tips for Healing from Liposuction for Lymphedema and Lipedema

Liposuction can be a valuable treatment for people with lymphedema. Lymphedema swelling is not just extra lymphatic fluid but can also be "accumulating adipose tissue and sometimes fibrosis" (Boyages et al., 2015). In the article "Liposuction for Advanced Lymphedema: A Multidisciplinary Approach for Complete Reduction of Arm and Leg Swelling," published in the *Annals of*

Surgical Oncology, Boyages et al. also detailed the results of a prospective clinical study of 104 patients and found that compression is a critical part of post-operative care for this operation. The size of your arm or leg will be smaller but compression garments still have to be worn because "ongoing reduction [is] maintained by continuous compression garment use" (2015).

How can we tell when liposuction of adipose tissue may be necessary for a patient with lymphedema? In the article "Liposuction Treatment of Lymphedema" published in *Seminars in Plastic Surgery*, Schaverien, Munnoch & Brorson explain why liposuction for lymphedema is performed, saying "excess volume without pitting means that adipose tissue is responsible for the swelling. Adipose tissue can be removed with liposuction. Conservative treatment and microsurgical reconstructions cannot do this" (2018).

Schaverien, Munnoch & Brorson also believe compression garment use is of utmost importance in the success of this surgery. The article says "garments are renewed 3 or 4 times during the first year. Two sets of … garments are always at the patient's disposal: one is worn while the other is washed. Thus, a garment is worn permanently, and treatment is interrupted only briefly when showering and, possibly, for formal social occasions." Bottom line: Schaverien, Munnoch & Brorson believe "it is essential that patients are compliant with compression garments preoperatively and agree to continuous wearing of compression garments following the surgery; non-compliance will lead to rebound increases in pitting edema" (2018).

Liposuction for lipedema focuses on removing diseased adipose tissue. In the article "Dilated Blood and Lymphatic Microvessels, Angiogenesis, Increased Macrophages, and Adipocyte Hypertrophy in Lipedema Thigh Skin and Fat Tissue," published in the *Journal of Obesity*, Al-Ghadban et al. found that "hypertrophic adipocytes, increased numbers of macrophages and blood vessels, and dilation of capillaries in thigh tissue of non-obese women with lipedema suggest inflammation, and angiogenesis occurs independent of obesity and demonstrates a role of altered vasculature in the manifestation of the disease" (2019).

Manual Lymphatic Drainage and compression garments are important parts of post-op care for lipedema liposuction surgery. The article "Liposuction in the Treatment of Lipedema: A Longitudinal Study," published in the *Archives of Plastic Surgery*, outlined results from "twenty-five patients who received 72 liposuction procedures for the treatment of lipedema." Dadras et al. shared that "new garments were measured 3 weeks after liposuction and after swelling had decreased, and manual lymphatic drainage was allowed after postoperative day 2" (2017). Another study that focused on older patients with lipedema recommended lymphatic drainage on a "regular basis, starting 2 weeks after liposuction" as well as "individual nonelastic flat knitted compression garments for a postsurgical period of 6 months." The patients also underwent a lower partial abdominoplasty and wore "a compression girdle for about 12 weeks" (Wollina et al., 2014).

In Shiffman & Di Giuseppe's book, *Liposuction: Principles and practice*, Cornely says "presurgical and postsurgical manual lymph drainage is indispensable. The postsurgical manual lymph drainage results in rapider healing and mobilization of the remaining tumescence solution out of the areas operated upon. Consistent wearing of a compression dressing for at least 8 weeks is recommended. If the compression dressing was worn for up to 16 weeks, clearly better results could be achieved compared with results from the usual short wearing periods of only 4 weeks." (2006, 333).

Your doctor knows your individual situation and will be able to give you information about the compression garments that are right for you.

A Few Tips for Healing from Abdominoplasty / Tummy Tuck

Yes, being slightly bent forward is a natural part of recovering from a tummy tuck. After three to four weeks you should feel like you are standing straighter. I have had good results adding a few minutes of low back massage to the lymphatic drainage massage sessions of my tummy tuck clients.

Some movement is good for healing from a tummy tuck, but more is not better. Dr. Gayoso recommends that his clients "pump their legs and walk as many times during the day as possible to prevent any blood clot formation" but "refrain from strenuous activities for a total of three months so as to preserve the internal corset-like effect of the operation" (Tummy Tuck: 8 Tips For A Successful Recovery, 2019).

Housework can interfere with achieving optimal results from a tummy tuck. ASAPS recommends that clients recovering from abdominoplasty "have lots of help at home.... If you have small children, you must put someone else totally in charge of their care for at least two weeks" (Tummy Tuck, 2018).

Abdominoplasty is different for men! Vidal et al. say "male patients tend to present less pleasing scars than women following abdominoplasty. The inguinal skin in men is thinner and more pigmented than the rest of the skin in the abdominal region. Differences in skin colour between both sides of the scar, along with a disparity in skin thickness, result in a suboptimal aesthetic outcome" (2017).

A Few Tips for Healing From A Facelift

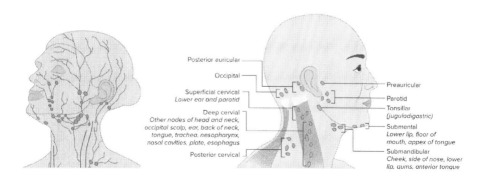

Sasada and Guest say their clients have told them "a wide-toothed comb will prevent you snagging the sutures as you comb your hair. Baby shampoo is much more comfortable to use post-operatively as it does not cause the wounds to sting. A child-sized toothbrush may be helpful as your mouth opening may be restricted for a few days after surgery" (2016). ASAPS recommends that clients recovering from a facelift can rest in a recliner, as "it is best for elevating the feet, knees and head. If you do not have a recliner, be sure to have lots of pillows available to prop up your head and knees." Clients should also select post-surgery outfits with tops that "open in front and do not have to be pulled over your head" (Facelift, 2018).

If you still have swelling a few months after surgery and your surgeon has cleared you for exercise, consider trying a few head and neck exercises. Moving the head and contracting your facial muscles moves fluids away from the swollen area and reduces adhesions. Neck exercises include lateral flexion, rotation and extension. Try it yourself with this video from the lymphoedema team at University College Hospital London: https://youtu.be/8SxmntTVVLs.

A Few Tips for Healing from Bilateral Eyelid Surgery

My first tip for healing from blepharoplasty is patience. I often find that after a week or two, my clients look much improved after their facelift but are still distressed about redness, bruising and swelling around their eyes. This is completely normal and will resolve. If you are really worried, there may be help for the bruising after eyelid surgery. In an article titled "The Efficacy of Intense Pulsed Light Therapy in Postoperative Recovery from Eyelid Surgery" published in *Plastic and Reconstructive Surgery*, Linkov et al. found that "in a series of patients who underwent eyelid surgery, intense pulsed light therapy decreased the degree of ecchymosis" (2016). If you find it difficult to completely close your eyes after surgery, ask your doctor if it is safe to wear a sleep mask to bed. This tip really helped one of my clients and improved her sleep.

A Few Tips for Healing after Facial Feminization Surgery

In the book *The Look of a Woman: Facial Feminization Surgery and the Aims of Trans-Medicine*, Eric Plemons says the patient "may need to suction saliva from her mouth because the throat pack placed during surgery will make it uncomfortable to swallow" and for a few days after surgery "she may need to manually stretch the muscles of her jaw" to keep them from clamping shut (2017).

A Few Tips for Healing from Double Jaw Surgery

Lauryn Evarts-Bosstick underwent double jaw surgery and shares her recovery tips in the post "My Corrective Double Jaw Surgery Experience" on her *Skinny Confidential* blog. She swears by lymphatic drainage! Read her post at https://www.theskinnyconfidential.com/corrective-double-jaw-surgery-experience.

A Few Tips for Healing After Liposuction

Wearing a compression garment will make your skin drier than usual. Foldi & Foldi state that "skin that is additionally burdened by compression therapy must be kept smooth and pliant and capable of bearing this burden." There are a few different ways you can help keep your skin moisturized while wearing compression. Foldi & Foldi recommend using soap-free cleansers like "showering oils" and applying moisturiser after bathing (Foldi & Foldi, 2012 p. 558). Healthy, hydrated and well-moisturized skin is important for everyone, especially after surgery. Choose a low pH lotion and remember that perfumed body lotions may actually dry the skin. Make sure your lotion is completely absorbed before you put on your garment. If you like scented lotion, consider making your own by combining a drop of a favorite floral or fruity essential oil into a palmful of lotion. Just for safety, only use a plain lotion approved by your plastic surgeon near your incision area.

Liposuction is different for men! Engler says "the skin and subcutaneous tissue tend to be particularly thick and dense (when compared with that of a woman). Because of this difference in skin thickness, an area of 'excess' may not be quite as thin postoperatively as would a similar area on a woman" (2000).

Sotelo-Paz recommends that her abdominal liposuction clients place a marble or cotton ball in their navel "so the belly button doesn't lose its shape" (2016). I have seen specially designed navel inserts for sale on social media sites. Ask your doctor before trying this. Do keep watch on the appearance of your belly button if you are wearing a compression garment on your abdominal area. Some women have found their belly button deviates to one side as a result of putting their garment on and pulling it to one side to latch the hooks of the garment.

Be sure to let your doctor know you have had liposuction if you are seeking treatment for uterine fibroids or adenomyosis. Zhao et al. found that "liposuction can increase the risk of skin burns in women with uterine fibroids or adenomyosis who desire sonographically guided HIFU therapy" (2014).

A Few Tips on Healing From Surgery After Massive Weight Loss

If you had surgery after a massive weight loss, watch

out for seromas. In the article "Liposuction Assisted Abdominoplasty: An Enhanced Abdominoplasty Technique" published in *Plastic and Reconstructive Surgery*, Brauman et al. say "seroma formation occurred much more commonly in massive weight loss patients" and comment that "it seems that weight loss results in the loss of fat but the supporting tissue, containing enlarged, numerous blood vessels, nerves and lymphatics, appears to have been retained. This could explain the preponderance for seroma formation" (2018). Using drains will help reduce the incidence of seroma (Janis et al., 2016).

A Few Tips on Healing After an Inner Thigh Lift

Swelling is a factor in thigh-lift operations. Olesen & Olesen say "the lymphatic system will usually clear away the excess fluid from the tissues. Rarely, the lymphatic ducts remain blocked and cause chronic swelling, which is most likely to happen when the inner thighs are lifted." This happens because "the main lymphatic drainage of the leg passes through the groin and is at risk for injury" (2005). In the article "Body Contouring by Combined Abdominoplasty and Medial Vertical Thigh Reduction: Experience of 14 Cases," published in the *Journal of Plastic, Reconstructive & Aesthetic Surgery*, Ellabban & Hart found that 28.6% of their clients "had trivial lower leg swelling which was treated conservatively by leg elevation, compression stockings and massage and eventually resolved" (2004).

How can you help in the healing process? In a thigh lift, "healing problems in this area are more common because of the likelihood of fecal and urinary contamination with subsequent infection." Olesen & Olesen recommend "in addition to using antibiotics, that you wash the entire operative area with soap and water, in the shower, following every bowel movement and urination" (2005).

A Few Tips on Healing From Fat Grafting for Gluteal Augmentation (BBL)

In the article "Experience With High-Volume Buttock Fat Transfer: A Report of 137 Cases," published in the *Aesthetic Surgery Journal*, Thomas Pane advises his clients "not to sit or lie on the buttocks for at least 7 days. Patients were encouraged to massage all liposuctioned areas, either at home or with the aid of massage therapists experienced in post-liposuction care." Pane says it "seems that the initial 'volume loss' is early postoperative swelling rather than reabsorption of significant amounts of fat." Some clients complain about persistent buttock dimples. Pane says "subcision and grafting . . . can be performed when patients present with dimples and seek improvement. Standard fat transfer techniques will improve most buttock dimples by increasing buttock volume, but dimples seldom resolve completely" (2019).

Family Wisdom

What are some ways you have healed your wounds in the past? Did your parents or grandparents have a home remedy that worked? Write that advice down here:

_____

_____

Want to learn more about how to heal your wounds? Physical Therapist Heather Flexer has a wealth of resources on wound healing at her Facebook page Better Wounds. Check it out at https://www.facebook.com/betterwounds.heatherflexer.

Beauty is an activity of the mind. – Thomas Aquinas

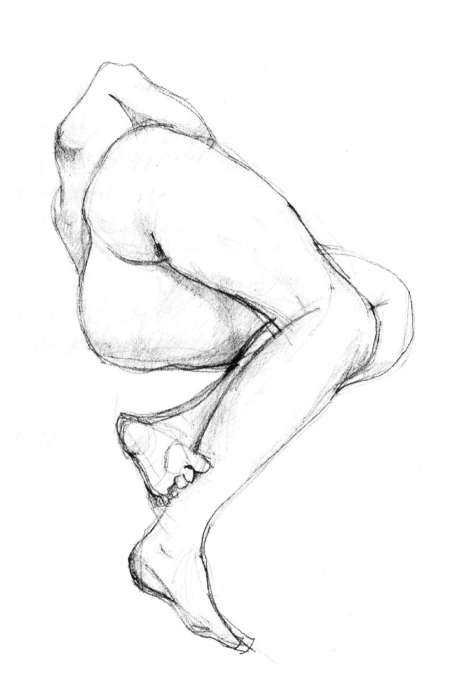

CHAPTER 7
GET BACK ON YOUR FEET

Exercise

Too much exercise is a big no-no in the days and weeks after surgery. Once your surgeon gives you the green light to exercise again, moving regularly is essential to long-term health.

In the first week, you may only be able to take short walks inside your home. No straining, bending over, or lifting! Moving around several times per day will reduce your risk for a blood clot. If you find that you just can't get motivated to move, consider taking entertainment devices out of your bedroom. This will encourage you to walk to the living room more often! Ask your surgeon if it is safe to perform one minute of ankle pumps (flexion and extension) once or twice per hour when you are awake to increase blood flow.

The second and third week, you may be able to walk for a short time outside, just up and down the street.

Between the fourth and sixth weeks, your doctor may allow you to participate in light exercise.

My clients who are athletes are often the toughest on themselves. Don't expect to go right back to your old workout at the gym. You must start slowly and build up to your pre-surgery level of fitness. In the study "The Effect of Detraining after a Period of Training on Cardiometabolic Health in Previously Sedentary Individuals," published in the *International Journal of Environmental Research and Public Health*, Nolan et al. found that after three months of exercising, "those people who subsequently detrained, the cardiometabolic health benefits were nearly completely reversed within one week of detraining" and "cessation of regular exercise rapidly abolished all training adaptations with one month of detraining" (2018). Be kind to your body and start again slowly.

Bed rest can also affect the body's health. In the study "Functional Impact of 10 Days of Bed Rest in Healthy Older Adults," published in the *Journals of Gerontology*, Kortebein et al. found "in healthy older adults, 10 days of bed rest results in a substantial loss of lower extremity strength, power, and aerobic capacity, and a reduction in physical activity" (2008).

If you need motivation to start exercising, research has found that using a pedometer may help. In a study titled "Using Pedometers to Increase Physical Activity and Improve Health: A Systematic Review" published in the *Journal of the American Medical Association*, Bravata et al. found that "pedometer users increased their physical activity by 26.9%" and "an important predictor of increased physical activity was having a step goal such as 10 000 steps per day" (2007).

Once you are allowed to exercise normally, there are a few exercises that can help reduce swelling, including:

- Gentle Yoga. Try this Lymphatic Flow Yoga Series with Shoosh Lettick Crotzer: https://youtu. be/8btp39n5luc or Lymphatic Yoga with Edely Wallace: https://lymphaticyoga.net
- Rebounding. Remember discovering the fun of jumping on a trampoline when you were a kid? A gentler version of that exercise can help move lymphatic fluid. Try gently bouncing on a rebounder—a small trampoline with a safety bar / handrail. The movement of the ankle and knee joints and the contraction and relaxation of the calf muscles help move lymphatic fluid out of the legs and feet. This may reduce swelling in your legs, ankles, and feet
- Swimming or water aerobics (usually patients aren't allowed to swim for at least a month after surgery)
- If you are experiencing swelling in the arms, consider incorporating a squishy stress ball in your workouts. Squeezing the ball will move the joints in your hand, giving your lymphatic system a boost

Taking Care of Your New Body

A word of caution if you have had liposuction: if you gain weight after the operation, it may settle in new parts of your body. In "Disharmonious Obesity Following Liposuction," Chapter 51 of the book *Liposuction Principles and Practice*, James E. Fulton Jr. and Farzin Kerendian describe "disharmonious obesity after liposuction" as occurring when "after removing one portion of the body's fat cells, the other fat cells may pick up the burden of fat storage" (2006, 342).

What does disharmonious obesity look like? Engler says "if fat is added, it will arrange itself in a different distribution throughout the body than it would have before the liposuction. For example, if, before surgery, a woman who gained a few pounds noted that most of it would go to her thighs and hips, then after surgery (i.e., liposuction of the thighs and hips), the fat will typically go to different areas, such as the stomach, chest, or arms." For men, Engler says, "just as the stomach, hips, and thighs are often treated together in women, the chest, stomach, and love handles are often treated together in men" (2000).

There is good news! In the Brazilian study "Liposuction Induces a Compensatory Increase of Visceral Fat Which is Effectively Counteracted by Physical Activity: a Randomized Trial," Benatti et al. found that "exercise training is capable of counteracting the liposuction induced compensatory growth of visceral fat in normal-weight women" and that there is a "protective effect of exercise training in preventing the visceral fat compensatory growth in response to liposuction." Study participants' exercise routines started two months after surgery and were tracked for four months. Workouts consisted of a five-minute warm-up "followed by strength exercises [eight exercises for the major muscle groups; one (during the first week as an adaptation training period) to three sets of eight to 12 repetitions maximum (RM) per exercise; 30 min/session] and by aerobic exercise on a treadmill (30–40 min/session) at an intensity corresponding to the respiratory compensation threshold [approximately 75% of the maximal oxygen uptake ($VO2_{max}$)] monitored using a heart rate monitor." There were no dietary restrictions (2012). I have put the webpage URL for this study in the back of the book. Print the study out and show it to your personal trainer if you would like to replicate the workouts tested in this study.

Walking is a good exercise to use when you begin getting fit again after surgery. If you had liposuction to your abdomen or torso area, consider walking barefoot on grass or the beach. You'll be surprised how much walking on an uneven surface activates your core muscles.

Using electrical muscle stimulation (EMS) when walking may be a good option for exercise after abdominal liposuction. Yes, some of those ab toning belts do have science to back their effectiveness. Similar devices are nicknamed Russian Stimulation due to their use by elite athletes in that country in the 20th century (Ward & Shkuratova, 2002).

Professionally, this modality is used by physical therapists when "traditional exercise is not possible due to injury or surgery ... as a means of maintaining muscular strength and minimizing atrophy due to immobilization" (Porcari, 2018). Certified Athletic Therapist Marina White shares that she uses EMS on her clients "to produce twitch muscle contractions to act like a pumping system to get the swelling out of the joint" (2017).

In a study titled "An 8-week Randomized Controlled Trial on the Effects of Brisk Walking, and Brisk Walking with Abdominal Electrical Stimulation on Anthropometric, Body Composition, and Self-Perception Measures in Sedentary Adult Women," published in *Psychology of Sport and Exercise*, subjects used an EMS device while walking briskly for thirty minutes on five days of each week for eight weeks. Anderson et al. say "walking + EMS could serve a protective function preventing an increase in umbilicus circumference [waist measurement]" (2006).

A few words of caution: make sure you have your surgeon's permission before you try an EMS device, especially if you have had a tummy tuck. These devices are regulated by the FDA. Learn more about potential risks at the FDA webpage on Electronic Muscle Stimulators at https://www.fda.gov/medicaldevices/productsandmedicalprocedures/homehealthandconsumer/consumerproducts/ucm142478.htm.

Whole-body vibration is another modality that may help strengthen muscles after surgery. In the paper "Vibration as an exercise modality: How it may work, and what its potential might be," published in the *European Journal of Applied Physiology*, Rittweger found "vibration training seems to improve muscle power, although the potential benefits over traditional forms of resistive exercise are still unclear. Vibration training also seems to improve balance in sub-populations prone to fall" (2010). Try sitting on a flat surface with just your feet on the vibration machine, then work up to standing or even performing exercises on the machine. As with any form of exercise, make sure it is okay with your surgeon before you try whole-body vibration.

Is non-surgery-related body pain limiting your ability to exercise? Finnish or infrared (IR) sauna may help. In the article "Clinical Effects of Regular Dry Sauna Bathing: A Systematic Review," published in *Evidence-Based Complementary and Alternative Medicine*, Hussain and Cohen say "saunas, either Finnish-style or infrared, may benefit people with rheumatic diseases such as fibromyalgia, rheumatoid arthritis, and ankylosing spondylitis, as well as patients with chronic fatigue and pain syndromes" as well as "improve exercise performance in athletes" (2018). In the study "Infrared Sauna in Patients with Rheumatoid Arthritis and Ankylosing Spondylitis," published in *Clinical Rheumatology*, patients were "treated for a period of 4 weeks, twice weekly, with eight IR sessions in the IR cabin (30 min at an ambient temperature of 55°C)" and authors recommend "patients should first experience a couple of trial sessions to see whether they achieve any clinical benefit prior to commencing a course of IR" (Oosterveld et al., 2009).

Sauna is a Northern European wellness practice widely practiced in Finland. I fondly remember my day spent exploring the saunas in the renowned Caracalla Therme in Baden-Baden, Germany. If you are looking for a way to enjoy sauna but your health club does not have one, portable infrared saunas are sold online.

"Everything has beauty, but not everyone sees it."
— Confucius

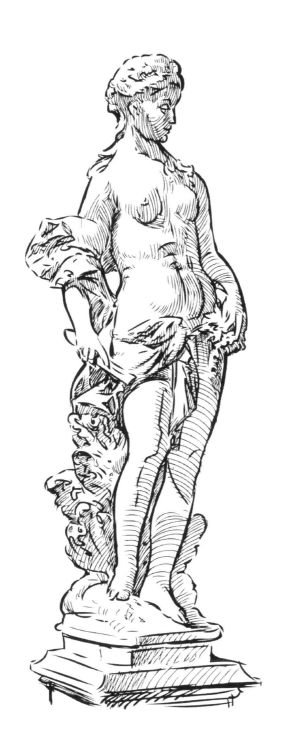

CHAPTER 8

FEEL HEALTHY INSIDE AND OUT

I felt a lot of anxiety when I was diagnosed with skin cancer on my face and scheduled for surgery. My husband and brother were the only people I told about the surgery before it happened. I didn't tell anyone else, not even my best friend. It's hard to explain why. I didn't want it to be a big deal and have to hear everyone's opinions on what was happening. I guess I wanted to wait to know that it was successful and then emerge a new, happier person to my family and friends.

That's not the advice I want to give to you! In the book *The Gifts of Imperfection*, Brené Brown shares that "one of the greatest barriers to connection is the cultural importance we place on 'going it alone.' Somehow we've come to equate success with not needing anyone" (2010, 20). I agree with Olesen & Olesen when they recommend that "no matter how independent you are, having an emotional support system increases your satisfaction" and "you'll be glad when they rally around during your recovery" (2005). We can be strong and still ask for help and support when we need it.

The desire to hide our plastic surgeries from others can also be cultural. In the book *Fat: The anthropology of an obsession*, Kulick & Meneley explain that "whereas cosmetic surgery in the US or Europe is still seen as a private matter, and one that is slightly embarrassing or at least socially awkward, in Brazil surgeries … are very public matters" (2005).

Post-Surgery Blues are Natural

Experiencing different feelings after surgery is normal. McNemar et al. remind their patients that "one common aftereffect of cosmetic surgery that you may not anticipate is a brief emotional letdown or depression." They say that "these feelings often surface about three days after surgery" and that "the emotional low may stem from metabolic changes in the body, fatigue, stress, or the frustration felt when results don't appear as quickly as hoped" (2006). Olesen & Olesen say "if you stay at home and are isolated from friends and co-workers, you may feel cut off from your normal environment, which can contribute to some level of temporary depression" (2005).

Getting a few days off to sit around and watch TV sounds so wonderful when we're busy at work, but it can make us feel stir-crazy when we're actually trapped on the couch. Kristina Robinson, the CEO of Curvy Gyals, shares some tips for handling feelings after plastic surgery in the video "Post Surgery Depression." Watch it at https://youtu.be/GcdqQPeH7O0.

Recovery from surgery can be a roller coaster of emotions, especially if people around us aren't fully supportive. If anything at all goes wrong with our recovery, it's all too easy to blame ourselves. We signed up for an "unnecessary surgery," didn't we? Recovering is hard enough as it is without also feeling guilt and a little regret as we are struggling with the healing process. What would it feel like to change the story of your surgery from "I am so vain, I did this to myself, I have only myself to blame" and instead think "I am on a journey to improve myself physically and emotionally and I am open to asking for help along the way"?

For many people, including myself, asking for help is difficult. Brené Brown wrote "for years, I placed value on being the helper in my family. I could help with a crisis or lend money or dispense advice. I was always happy to help others, but I would have never called my siblings to ask them for help.... I understand how I derived self-worth from never needing help and always offering it" (2010, 21). You're not alone in wanting to depend only on yourself. If your recovery is feeling too difficult, it's okay to rely on close friends and family while you are healing.

Let's play around with this! Use these prompts, or, even better, use a sheet of paper and list your responses to "I could ask (name) for (something you want/need)."

I could ask _____ for _____

I could ask _____ for _____

I could ask _____ for _____

I could ask _____ for _____

I could ask _____ for _____

I could ask _____ for _____

Keeping a Post-Surgery Journal

Another way to stay optimistic during your recovery is to keep a journal. Schafer recommends that his patients keep a journal starting the day after their surgery and "every day, look for improvements, no matter how slight, and enter them into your diary. When you start to feel like you're not progressing, go back and read a few pages" (2011). You can use the sample diary in the back of this book or create your own.

What to Have on Hand While Recovering

If you're reading this before surgery, I recommend buying Peggy Huddleston's *Prepare for Surgery, Heal Faster* book. Huddleston's method of focusing on positive imagery has resulted in patients reducing their anxiety levels before surgery, using less pain medication, and recovering faster after their operation. Huddleston recommends that before surgery you visualize your healing, organize a support group, and use healing statements. The power of focusing on personalized positive imagery has been documented in research studies at the Lahey Clinic (Tufts University Medical School), New England Baptist Hospital (Tufts University Medical School) and Beth Israel Deaconess Medical Center (Harvard Medical School). I highly recommend talking with your surgeon and anesthetist about incorporating healing statements into your surgery experience.

After my reconstructive surgery, I remember wandering around in a daze at the drug store after being released from the hospital, trying to buy meal replacement drinks while my prescription was being filled. Luckily my friend Elyssa was there to drive me home! Don't be like me—plan ahead.

Post-surgery shopping list

- ▶ Loose, easy on/off clothing in dark colors
- ▶ If you enjoy essential oils, your favorite lavender, rose, orange/lemon, geranium, or frankincense essential oil and a diffuser
- ▶ Laxative (if recommended by physician) and chewing gum and Coffee or Tea
- ▶ Maxi pads (cost-effective option for absorbing bodily fluids) or wound dressings
- ▶ Dog potty-training pads (protect your bed or chair from bodily fluids)

- ▶ Baby wipes (for in between showers)
- ▶ Slip-on shoes/slippers
- ▶ Urine funnel
- ▶ Foot stool
- ▶ Grabbing tool
- ▶ First aid kit and bandages
- ▶ Large hand mirror (to see incisions on your side or back)
- ▶ Plastic mattress cover (makes sliding over and getting up from bed easier)
- ▶ Ironing board to use as an extra table when you can't bend down easily
- ▶ Shower Chair—How to use a Shower chair video https://youtu.be/lCefLm0-QOM
- ▶ Walker
- ▶ BBL pillow if you have had BBL surgery
- ▶ Refrigerator stocked with easy to prepare, easy to eat foods. A tummy tuck client introduced me to grocery delivery service, a great option for getting fresh food delivered to your home when you cannot make it to the store.

ASAPS recommends that clients recovering from abdominoplasty keep food and toiletries at hip level and keep medications on the nightstand, with a pill organizer and written medication schedule (Tummy Tuck, 2018).

Why is chewing gum on the list? According to the study "A Systematic Review of the Efficacy of Gum Chewing for the Amelioration of Postoperative Ileus" published in *Digestive Surgery*, de Castro et al. found that "trials have shown promising results for the efficacy of gum chewing for the amelioration of postoperative ileus [a temporary condition where the bowels are unable to function and move feces out of the body]" and "this meta-analysis shows a favorable effect of gum chewing on time to flatus and defecation." What does that mean? Ask your surgeon if you are allowed to chew gum after your surgery. By fooling the body into thinking you are eating, it may reactivate your digestive system and help you to poop (2008).

Drinking caffeine may have a similar positive effect! According to the study "Effect of Caffeine Intake on Postoperative Ileus: A Systematic Review and Meta-Analysis" published in *Digestive Surgery*, Gkegkes et al. found that the "postoperative administration of coffee improves bowel motility reducing the time to first bowel movement, the time to first flatus and to defecation" (Gkegkes et al, 2019).

How to Take The Focus Off Your Surgery

Olesen & Olesen warn their clients to "be prepared for lots of feedback from your friends and family" and point out that "many friends are more focused on our flaws than our progress when they see us after plastic surgery, but that these are nonmedical opinions" (2005).

How can you handle the reactions of acquaintances? If you want to keep the topic of conversation off your surgery, Engler recommends that before surgery you consider "getting exactly what other people think they're seeing—a new haircut, color or style, new glasses, and/or some new clothes" (2000).

What about that little voice in your own head? Sometimes the days and weeks after surgery can feel overwhelming and our inner voice can be very judgmental. Take comfort—you are not alone.

Society would have us believe that everyone who makes an appointment to see a plastic surgeon is hopelessly vain. Research has proven otherwise. In Chapter 55 of Liposuction Principles and Practice, "Psychology and Quality of Life of Patients Undergoing Liposuction Surgery," Sattler et al. found that "between the two extremes of self-neglect versus overconcern and negative versus beautified self-image there are a wide range of people with a so-called normal concern and perception of their appearance. These are people who care for themselves without exaggeration and have a realistic view of their outer appearance. They are the peer group for cosmetic medicine." They cite a study of three hundred patients undergoing liposuction surgery that found "patients undergoing liposuction are in most cases happy with the treatment and experience positive effects for body, mind and social interactions" (Shiffman & Di Giuseppe 2006, 364–365).

Knowing this, what would happen if you changed the topic of inner conversation, just for a while, to something more pleasant?

Let's play around with this! Just like the song "My Favorite Things" from The Sound of Music, use these prompts, or, even better, use a sheet of paper and list your answer to the question "What are a few of my favorite things?" Come back to the list when you need a little boost.

_____

_____

_____

_____

How to Know That You Are Healing

In *Prepare for Surgery, Heal Faster*, Peggy Huddleston recommends using positive imagery to keep your focus on a full recovery. She explains how to set an image of how you will feel immediately after surgery, midway through healing and when you are fully recovered. When we are living life day to day, sometimes it is hard to recognize that our body is actually healing. Having an image in mind of what it will feel like to be fully recovered can guide us.

For me, being fully recovered after my reconstructive surgery meant running five miles on a treadmill at the gym. I remember getting off the treadmill that day feeling so happy that I was able to be active again!

Using a body scan meditation also helped me to focus on how I was healing after a bad ankle sprain. I was focused on babying my ankle and feeling disappointed in my lack of progress toward recovery. Taking time to check in with what my body was feeling in that moment helped me to realize that I no longer had pain in my ankle while at rest. This realization helped me become more optimistic about my recovery.

Try a body scan meditation for yourself at https://health. ucsd.edu/specialties/mindfulness/programs/mbsr/ pages/audio.aspx.

Planning for Life After Surgery: Dimensions of Positive Health

In our parents' day, people were either healthy or they were sick. Now we know that there are many dimensions of wellness, including physical, mental, spiritual, emotional, and social. I want to share a rather new concept of health that comes to us from the Netherlands.

Positive Health can be defined as "the ability to adapt and to self manage, in the face of social, physical and emotional challenges," according to the article "How Should We Define Health?" by Huber et al. published in the *British Medical Journal* in 2011. In a study published in the same journal in 2016, Huber et al. listed six dimensions of positive health:

* Bodily functions include physical functioning of our body, complaints, pain, and energy levels
* Mental functions and perception include cognitive functioning, our emotional state, self-respect, self-management and resilience
* Spiritual/existential dimension includes a sense of meaning/meaningfulness, striving for aims/ideals, and acceptance
* Quality of life includes well-being, experiencing happiness, enjoyment, a zest for life, and sense of balance
* Social and societal participation includes social and communicative skills, meaningful relationships, our social contacts, the feeling of being accepted, community involvement, and meaningful work
* Daily functioning includes being able to complete the activities of daily living and the ability to work

For many people, the reason they want plastic surgery is to improve a flaw that embarrasses them or to restore their sense of looking like the person they feel like on the inside. I encourage you to use the newfound confidence you feel after plastic surgery to foster your relationships and sense of connection with your community. What type of connection am I talking about? Brené Brown defines connection as "the energy that exists between people when they feel seen, heard, and valued; when they can give and receive without judgment; and when they derive sustenance and strength from the relationship" (2010).

In the book *Lost Connections: Uncovering the Real Causes of Depression—and the Unexpected Solutions*, Johann Hari quotes neuroscience researcher John Cacioppo: "Loneliness isn't the physical absence of other people.… It's the sense that you're not sharing anything that matters with anyone else. If you have lots of people around you—perhaps even a husband or wife, or a family, or a busy workplace—but you don't share anything that matters with them, then you'll still be lonely" (2018).

For many of my clients, embarrassment over their body limited their ability to foster connection through participation in physical and social activities. How can you adjust to and celebrate your new body? Here are a few ideas.

Volunteering or Joining Clubs

Can you let your enjoyment of the results of plastic surgery inspire you to be more active in your community? Olesen

& Olesen recommend their clients "join a book club or extension course" and "add some volunteer activities to your routine" (2005). In the book *The Stress Management Workbook: De-stress in 10 Minutes or Less*, Ruth C. White, a stress management and mental wellness expert, agrees: "The social connection that is associated with volunteering has significant positive impacts on your mental health and well-being and can lower your stress levels. Think about what change you want to see in the world and help an organization work toward that change. Giving to others may be altruistic, but it also feels good. It makes you feel useful, keeps you connected to something bigger than yourself, and puts your life in perspective" (2018).

Focusing on Positive Social Relationships

White also predicts that by "focusing on the positive aspects of life, you will feel better and subsequently relieve some stress. Spend a minute thinking about how to compliment a friend or family member and send some positivity their way. You'll find it reflected back at you, whether through a direct compliment or simply thinking about how lucky you are to have a loved one, family, or friends" (2018). Cacioppo also said "to end loneliness, you need other people—plus something else. You also need ... to feel you are sharing something with the other person, or the group, that is meaningful to both of you. You have to be in it together—and 'it' can be anything that you both think has meaning and value" (Hari, 2018).

Ways I Can Make Connections in my Community:

_____

_____

_____

Reconnect With Yourself

Healing from surgery can be an excellent time to discover meditation or rededicate yourself to a mindfulness practice. Can't get out of the house to join a meditation group? The Mindful Awareness Research Center at UCLA has a selection of six-week online courses you can try. Find out more at https://www.uclahealth.org/marc/online-classes.

Positive Health with Chronic Illness

Some of my clients have plastic surgery to improve their symptoms but still have the chronic diseases of lymphedema or lipedema. Interestingly, Huber et al. found that "having a chronic disease was itself independently related to a decrease in the value placed on bodily functions and an increase in the value awarded to the spiritual/existential dimension" (2016). Focusing more on building resilience and the ability to adapt to challenges as well as finding meaning through spirituality may be a path to positive health if you have a chronic illness.

Your Personal Self-Care Checklist

What kinds of activities would have to be on your personal self-care checklist to achieve Positive Health? I need regular exercise to keep my physical health excellent, regular massages to reduce body pain, meditation to keep me feeling balanced, meaningful work, and time spent with friends. I also have my limits. I can't be at my best when I have less than six hours of sleep at night or am on the go for more than ten hours a day. White recommends we write down our limits and "return to them when we feel stressed and need to be reminded of our limits. I need hours of sleep every night. I need to eat every few hours. I need to drink glasses of water each day. I need social interactions every day. I need minutes of exercise per day. I need minutes of alone time every day. I need minutes to meditate or pray. I need minutes to do nothing" (2018).

My Self-Care Checklist:

_____

_____

_____

_____

Final Thought

How can we adapt and self-manage when life's little emergencies get in the way of our plans? Like the Aesop's

Fable teaches us, a reed can bend in the wind but a tree cannot. How can you "bend in the wind" when life doesn't go your way?

"The most beautiful people we have known are those who have known defeat, known suffering, known struggle, known loss, and have found their way out of the depths. These persons have an appreciation, a sensitivity, and an understanding of life that fills them with compassion, gentleness, and a deep loving concern. Beautiful people do not just happen." — Elisabeth Kübler-Ross

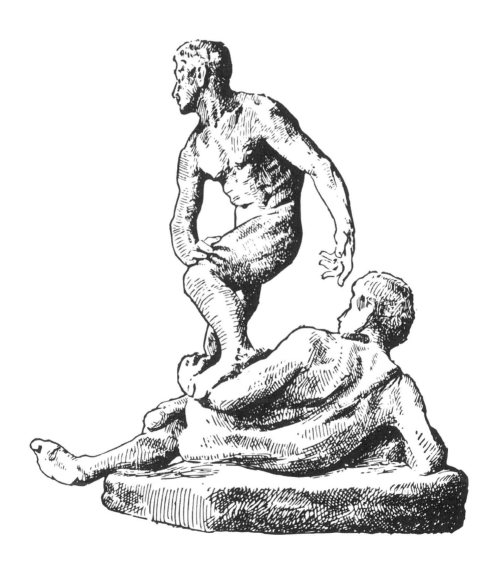

CONCLUSION

I hope this whirlwind tour through my plastic surgery recovery rules has given you the resources and confidence to discuss your healing plan with your plastic surgeon.

Remember to:

- Follow Doctor's Orders
- Reduce Swelling
- Reduce Bruising
- Improve Scars and Fibrosis
- Support Wound Healing
- Get Back on Your Feet and
- Feel Healthy Inside and Out!

Let me know your tips for healing from plastic surgery and follow me on social media for more tips:

Facebook: @PlasticSurgeryRecoveryHandbook

Instagram: @PlasticSurgeryRecoveryHandbook

Twitter: @KathleenLisson

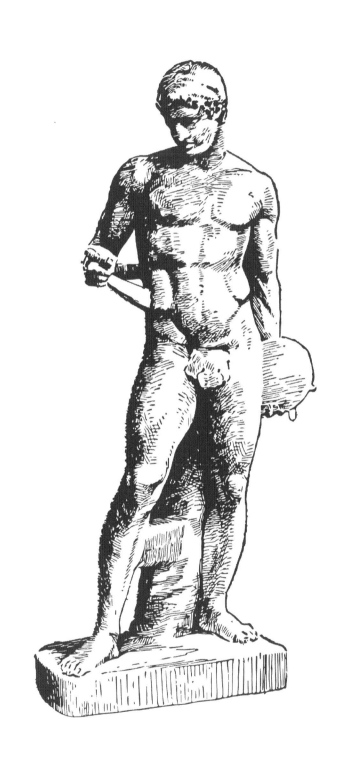

BIBLIOGRAPHY

6 Best Fixes for Pain and Swelling in Your Feet and Ankles. (2016, July 19). Retrieved from https://health.clevelandclinic.org/2016/06/6-best-ways-relieve-swollen-feet-ankles-home.

Ablon G. (2018). Phototherapy with light emitting diodes: Treating a broad range of medical and aesthetic conditions in dermatology. *Journal of Clinical and Aesthetic Dermatology*, 11(2), 21–27. Retrieved from https://www.ncbi.nlm.nih.gov/pmc/articles/PMC5843358/pdf/jcad_11_2_21.pdf.

Al-Ghadban S., Cromer W., Allen M., et al. Dilated blood and lymphatic microvessels, angiogenesis, increased macrophages, and adipocyte hypertrophy in lipedema thigh skin and fat tissue. *Journal of Obesity*, vol. 2019, Article ID 8747461, 10 pages. https://doi.org/10.1155/2019/8747461. Retrieved from https://www.hindawi.com/journals/jobe/2019/8747461/abs.

Alser, O. H., & Goutos, I. (2018). The evidence behind the use of platelet-rich plasma (PRP) in scar management: a literature review. *Scars, burns & healing*, 4, 2059513118808773. doi:10.1177/2059513118808773 Retrieved from: https://www.ncbi.nlm.nih.gov/pmc/articles/PMC6243404/

Anderson, A.G., Murphy, M.H., Murtagh, E., & Nevill, A. (2006). An 8-week randomized controlled trial on the effects of brisk walking, and brisk walking with abdominal electrical stimulation on anthropometric, body composition, and self-perception measures in sedentary adult women. *Psychology of Sport and Exercise*, 7, 437–451. Retrieved from https://doi.org/10.1016/j.psychsport.2006.04.003.

Anderson, K., & Hamm, R. L. (2014). Factors that impair wound healing. *Journal of the American College of Clinical Wound Specialists*, 4(4), 84–91. doi:10.1016/j.jccw.2014.03.001 Retrieved from https://www.ncbi.nlm.nih.gov/pmc/articles/PMC4495737.

Arno, A. I., Gauglitz, G. G., Barret, J. P., & Jeschke, M. G. (2014). Up-to-date approach to manage keloids and hypertrophic scars: a useful guide. *Burns: Journal of the International Society for Burn Injuries*, 40(7), 1255–66. Retrieved from https://www.ncbi.nlm.nih.gov/pmc/articles/PMC4186912.

Ashforth, K., Morgner, S., & Vanhoose, L. (2011). A new treatment for soft tissue fibrosis in the breast. *Journal of Lymphoedema*, 6, 42–46. Retrieved from https://www.researchgate.net/publication/281656383_A_new_treatment_for_soft_tissue_fibrosis_in_the_breast.

Atkinson J, McKenna K, Barnett A, McGrath D, & Rudd M. (2005). A randomized, controlled trial to determine the efficacy of paper tape in preventing hypertrophic scar formation in surgical incisions that traverse Langer's skin tension lines. *Plastic and Reconstructive Surgery*, 116(6), 1648–56. Retrieved from https://www.ncbi.nlm.nih.gov/pubmed/16267427.

Bae, H., & Kim, H. J. (2013). Clinical outcomes of extracorporeal shock wave therapy in patients with secondary lymphedema: a pilot study. *Annals of rehabilitation medicine*, 37(2), 229–234. doi:10.5535/arm.2013.37.2.229. Retrieved from: https://www.ncbi.nlm.nih.gov/pmc/articles/PMC3660484/

Bellini, E., Grieco, M. P., & Raposio, E. (2017). A journey through liposuction and liposculture: Review. *Annals of medicine and surgery* 24, 53–60. doi:10.1016/j.amsu.2017.10.024 Retrieved from https://www.ncbi.nlm.nih.gov/pmc/articles/PMC5681335.

Benatti, F., Solis, M., Artioli, G., Montag, E., Painelli, V., Saito,

F., Baptista, L., … & Lancha, A. Jr. (2012). Liposuction induces a compensatory increase of visceral fat which is effectively counteracted by physical activity: A randomized trial. *Journal of Clinical Endocrinology & Metabolism*, 97(7), 2388–95, doi:10.1210/jc.2012-1012. Retrieved from https://academic.oup.com/jcem/article/97/7/2388/2834256.

Block Therapy (2019). Retrieved from https://blocktherapy.com/about/

Boyages, J., Kastanias, K., Koelmeyer, L. A., Winch, C. J., Lam, T. C., Sherman, K. A., … & Mackie, H. (2015). Liposuction for advanced lymphedema: A multidisciplinary approach for complete reduction of arm and leg swelling. *Annals of surgical oncology*, 22 Suppl 3, 1263–70. doi:10.1245/s10434-015-4700-3 Retrieved from https://www.ncbi.nlm.nih.gov/pmc/articles/PMC4686553.

Brauman, D., van der Hulst, R., & van der Lei, B. (2018). Liposuction assisted abdominoplasty: An enhanced abdominoplasty technique. *Plastic and reconstructive surgery. Global open*, 6(9), e1940. doi:10.1097/GOX.0000000000001940 Retrieved from https://www.ncbi.nlm.nih.gov/pmc/articles/PMC6191222.

Bravata, D.M., Smith-Spangler, C., Sundaram, V., et al. (2007). Using pedometers to increase physical activity and improve health: A systematic review. *JAMA: The Journal of the American Medical Association*, 298(19), 2296–2304. doi:10.1001/jama.298.19.2296. Retrieved from https://jamanetwork.com/journals/jama/article-abstract/209526.

Brown, B. (2010). *The gifts of imperfection*. Hazelden Publishing.

Bylka, W., Znajdek-Awiżeń, P., Studzińska-Sroka, E., & Brzezińska, M. (2013). *Centella asiatica in cosmetology. Postepy Dermatologii i Alergologii [Advances in Dermatology and Allergology]*, 30(1), 46–9. Retrieved from https://www.ncbi.nlm.nih.gov/pmc/articles/PMC3834700.

Care Instructions (n.d.). Retrieved from: https://marenagroup.com/about/care/

Caring for Your Jackson-Pratt Drain (2019, Feb. 1). Retrieved from https://www.mskcc.org/cancer-care/patient-education/caring-your-jackson-pratt-drai

Carr, A. C., & Maggini, S. (2017). Vitamin C and immune function. *Nutrients*, 9(11), 1211. doi:10.3390/nu9111211. Retrieved from https://www.ncbi.nlm.nih.gov/pmc/articles/PMC5707683.

Casas, L. & DePilo, P. (1999). Manual lymphatic drainage therapy: An integral component of postoperative care in plastic surgery patients. *Proceedings of The First Annual Conference of the American Society of Lymphology*. 1999 Aug. Chicago. Retrieved from http://www.serenebodyworks.net/wp-content/uploads/2018/03/MLD-An-integral-Component-of-Postoperative-Care.pdf.

Chughtai, M., Newman, J. M., Sultan, A. A., Samuel, L. T., Rabin, J., Khlopas, A., … & Mont, M. A. (2019). Astym® therapy: a systematic review. *Annals of Translational Medicine*, 7(4), 70. doi:10.21037/atm.2018.11.49 Retrieved from https://www.ncbi.nlm.nih.gov/pmc/articles/PMC6409241.

Courtney, R. (2009). The functions of breathing and its dysfunctions and their relationship to breathing therapy. *International Journal of Osteopathic Medicine*, 12(3), 78–85. https://doi.org/10.1016/j.ijosm.2009.04.002 Retrieved from https://www.researchgate.net/publication/228637154_The_functions_of_breathing_and_its_dysfunctions_and_their_relationship_to_breathing_therapy.

Dadras, M., Mallinger, P. J., Corterier, C. C., Theodosiadi, S., & Ghods, M. (2017). Liposuction in the treatment of lipedema: A longitudinal study. *Archives of Plastic Surgery*, 44(4), 324–331.

doi:10.5999/aps.2017.44.4.324 Retrieved from https://www.ncbi. nlm.nih.gov/pmc/articles/PMC5533060.

Dayan, S. (2007). *Instant Beauty*. New York, NY: Hatherleigh Press.

de Castro, S. M. M., van den Esschert, J. W., van Heek, N. T., Dalhuisen, S., Koelemay, M. J. W., Busch, O. R. C., & Gouma, D. J. (2008). A systematic review of the efficacy of gum chewing for the amelioration of postoperative ileus. *Digestive Surgery*, 2008(25), 39–45. doi: 10.1159/000117822.

Direction Of Use And Care (n.d.). Retrieved from: https://www. isavela.com/pages/helpful-info/care-instructions.html

di Summa, P. G., Wettstein, R., Erba, P., et al. Scar asymmetry after abdominoplasty: The unexpected role of seroma. *Annals of Plastic Surgery*, 2013(71), 461 Retrieved from https://journals.lww.com/ annalsplasticsurgery/Abstract/2013/11000/Scar_Asymmetry_ After_Abdominoplasty__The.7.aspx.

Dixit, V. V., & Wagh, M. S. (2013). Unfavourable outcomes of liposuction and their management. *Indian Journal of Plastic Surgery*, 46(2), 377–92. Retrieved from https://www.ncbi.nlm.nih.gov/pmc/ articles/PMC3901919.

Donec, V. & Kriščiūnas, A. (2014). The effectiveness of Kinesio Taping® after total knee replacement in early postoperative rehabilitation period: A randomized clinical trial. *European Journal of Physical and Rehabilitation Medicine*, 50(4), 363–71. Retrieved from https://kinesiocourse.ru/files/mejdunaresled/2014/kttotalkn. pdf.

Doughty, D. B. Preventing and managing surgical wound dehiscence. *Advances in Skin & Wound Care*, 18(6), 319–322. Retrieved from https://insights.ovid.com/pubmed?pmid=16096397.

Ebert, J.R., Joss, B., Jardine, B., & Wood, D. J. (2013). Randomized trial investigating the efficacy of manual lymphatic drainage to improve early outcome after total knee arthroplasty. Archives of Physical Medicine and Rehabilitation, 94(11), 2103–11. Retrieved from https://www.archives-pmr.org/article/S0003-9993(13)00461-9/fulltext.

Ellabban, M.G. & Hart, N.B. (2004). Body contouring by combined abdominoplasty and medial vertical thigh reduction: Experience of 14 cases. *British Journal of Plastic Surgery*, 57(3), 222 – 227. Retrieved from https://www.jprasurg.com/article/S0007-1226(03)00585-X/fulltext.

Engler, A. M. (2000). *Bodysculpture: Plastic surgery of the body for men and women*. New York: Hudson Publishing.

FAQ (2019). Retrieved from https://www.bonitoandcompany.com/pages/faq.

Facelift (2018). Retrieved from https://www.smartbeautyguide.com/procedures/head-face/facelift.

Földi, E., Földi, M., (eds) (2012) *Textbook of lymphology*. Munich: Urban & Fischer.

Frequently Asked Questions (n.d.). Retrieved from: http://www.clearpointmedical.com/en/frequently-asked-questions-compression-wear.aspx

Fu, X., Dong, J., Wang, S., Yan, M., & Yao, M. (2019). Advances in the treatment of traumatic scars with laser, intense pulsed light, radiofrequency, and ultrasound. *Burns & Trauma*, 7, 1. doi:10.1186/s41038-018-0141-0. Retrieved from https://www.ncbi.nlm.nih.gov/pmc/articles/PMC6350396.

Garment Care (2017). Retrieved from https://www.wearease.com/pages/garment-care.

Garment Care (n.d.). Retrieved from https://solideaus.com/pages/garment-care.

Gasbarro, V., Bartoletti, R., Tsolaki, E., Sileno, S., Agnati, M., Coen, M., Conti, M., Bertaccini, (2006). Role of HIVAMAT ® 200 (deep oscillation) in the treatment of the lymphedema of the limbs. European Journal of Lymphology and Related Problems. 16(48). Retrieved from: https://www.eurolymphology.org/JOURNAL/Vol16-N48-2006.pdf

General Product Information & FAQs (n.d.). Retrieved from http://www.therapygarments.com/far-infrared-cellulite-clothing.html.

Gkegkes I, D, Minis E, E, Iavazzo C: Effect of Caffeine Intake on Postoperative Ileus: A Systematic Review and Meta-Analysis. Dig Surg 2019. doi: 10.1159/000496431 Retrieved from: https://www.karger.com/Article/FullText/496431#

Gouin, J. P., & Kiecolt-Glaser, J. K. (2012). The impact of psychological stress on wound healing: Methods and mechanisms. *Critical Care Nursing Clinics of North America*, 24(2), 201–13. Retrieved from https://www.ncbi.nlm.nih.gov/pmc/articles/PMC3775570.

Gott, F.H. & Ly, K. & Piller, N. & Mangio, A. (2018). Negative pressure therapy in the management of lymphoedema. *Journal of Lymphoedema*. 13. 43-48.

Guarneri, M. (2017). *108 pearls to awaken your healing potential: A cardiologist translates the science of health and healing into practice*. Carlsbad, CA: Hay House, Inc.

Hamblin M. R. (2017). Mechanisms and applications of the anti-inflammatory effects of photobiomodulation. *AIMS Biophysics*,

4(3), 337–361. Retrieved from https://www.ncbi.nlm.nih.gov/pmc/articles/PMC5523874.

Hamman, M. S., & Goldman, M. P. (2013). Minimizing bruising following fillers and other cosmetic injectables. *Journal of Clinical and Aesthetic Dermatology*, 6(8), 16–18. Retrieved from https://www.ncbi.nlm.nih.gov/pmc/articles/PMC3760599.

Hari, J. (2018). *Lost connections: Uncovering the real causes of depression—And the unexpected solutions*. Bloomsbury.

Healing Without Scars (2018, Nov. 7). Retrieved from https://hsci.harvard.edu/news/healing-without-scars.

Home Care for Your Wound Drain. (n.d.). Retrieved from https://patienteducation.osumc.edu/Documents/HomeCareWoundDrain.pdf.

How to Videos & Care (n.d.). Retrieved from: https://contemporarydesigninc.com/how-to-videos/

Huber, M., Knottnerus, J., Green, L., Horst, H., Jadad, A., Kromhout, D., … & Smid, H. How should we define health? BMJ, 2011(343), d4163. doi: 10.1136/bmj.d4163. Retrieved from https://www.bmj.com/content/343/bmj.d4163.

Huber, M., van Vliet, M., Giezenberg, M., B. Winkens, Y. Heerkens, P. C. Dagnelie, & J. A. Knottnerus. Towards a "patient-centred" operationalisation of the new dynamic concept of health: A mixed methods study. *BMJ Open* 2016;5:e010091. doi:10.1136/bmjopen-2015- 010091. Retrieved from http://www.louisbolk.org/downloads/3108.pdf.

Husain, T., Salgado, C., Mundra, L., Perez, C., AlQattan, H., Bustillo, E., … & Garri, J. (2019). Abdominal etching: Surgical technique and outcomes, *Plastic and Reconstructive Surgery*, 143(4), 1051–1060.

doi: 10.1097/PRS.0000000000005486. Retrieved from https://journals.lww.com/plasreconsurg/Fulltext/2019/04000/Abdominal_Etching__Surgical_Technique_and_Outcomes.15.aspx.

Hussain J. & Cohen M. (2018) Clinical effects of regular dry sauna bathing: A systematic review. *Evidence-Based Complementary and Alternative Medicine*, vol. 2018, Article ID 1857413, 30 pages. doi:10.1155/2018/1857413. Retrieved from https://www.hindawi.com/journals/ecam/2018/1857413/cta.

Instrument Assisted Soft Tissue Mobilisation (IASTM). (2019). Retrieved from http://www.ovmc-eorh.com/programs-and-services/physical-therapy/iastm.asp.

Janis, J. E., Khansa, L., & Khansa, I. (2016). Strategies for postoperative seroma prevention: a systematic review. *Plastic and Reconstructive Surgery*, 138(1), 240–252. Retrieved from https://journals.lww.com/plasreconsurg/Abstract/2016/07000/Strategies_for_Postoperative_Seroma_Prevention___A.41.aspx

Kiecolt-Glaser, J. K., Loving, T. J., Stowell, J. R., Malarkey, W. B., Lemeshow, S., Dickinson, S. L, & Glaser, R. (2005). Hostile marital interactions, proinflammatory cytokine production, and wound healing. Archives of General Psychiatry. 62(12), 1377–84. Retrieved from https://www.ncbi.nlm.nih.gov/pubmed/16330726

Klose, G. (2010). *Compression Bandaging for Lymphedema Management*. Neuwied, Germany: Lohmann & Rauscher.

Klose, G. (2014 Oct. 1) How manual lymph drainage certification will change your massage practice. Retrieved from https://www.massagemag.com/how-manual-lymph-drainage-certification-will-change-your-massage-practice-27028.

Knobloch, K., Joest, B., Krämer, R., & Vogt, P. M. (2013). Cellulite and focused extracorporeal shockwave therapy for non-invasive body contouring: a randomized trial. *Dermatology and therapy*, 3(2), 143–155. doi:10.1007/s13555-013-0039-5. Retrieved from: https://www.ncbi.nlm.nih.gov/pmc/articles/PMC3889306/

Komprex (n.d.). Retrieved from https://www.lohmann-rauscher. com/us-en/products/compression-therapy/padding-foam/ komprex.

Kortebein, P., Symons, T., Ferrando, A., Paddon-Jones, D., Ronsen, O., Protas, E., … & Evans, W. (2008). Functional impact of 10 days of bed rest in healthy older adults. *Journals of Gerontology: Series A*, 63(10), 1076–1081. doi: 10.1093/gerona/63.10.1076. Retrieved from https://academic.oup.com/biomedgerontology/ article/63/10/1076/559225.

Kulick, D., & Meneley, A. (2005). *Fat: The anthropology of an obsession*. New York: Jeremy P. Tarcher/Penguin.

Laser Therapy for Lymphedema. (2012, Sept. 17). Retrieved from https://www.breastcancer.org/treatment/lymphedema/treatments/ laser.

Levine, J. (2004). Non-exercise activity thermogenesis (Neat). *Nutrition Reviews*, 62(suppl_2), S82–S97. doi: 10.1111/j.1753-4887.2004.tb00094.x. Retrieved from https://academic.oup.com/ nutritionreviews/article-abstract/62/suppl_2/S82/1812445.

Linkov, G., Lam, V. B., & Wulc, A. E. (2016). The efficacy of intense pulsed light therapy in postoperative recovery from eyelid surgery. *Plastic and Reconstructive Surgery*, 137(5), 783e-789e. Retrieved from https://journals.lww.com/plasreconsurg/ Abstract/2016/05000/The_Efficacy_of_Intense_Pulsed_Light_ Therapy_in.10.aspx.

Liposuction (2018). Retrieved from https://www.smartbeautyguide. com/procedures/body/liposuction/

McNemar, T., Salzberg, C. A., & Seidel, S. (2006). *Breast augmentation and body contouring*. Omaha, NE: Addicus Books.

MacKay, D. & Miller, A. L. (2003). Nutritional support for wound healing. Alternative Medicine Review, 8(4), 359–377. Retrieved from http://archive.foundationalmedicinereview.com/publications/8/4/359.pdf.

Mayrovitz, H. N. & Yzer, J. A. (2017). Local skin cooling as an aid to the management of patients with breast cancer related lymphedema and fibrosis of the arm or breast. *Lymphology*, 50(2), 56–66. Retrieved from https://journals.uair.arizona.edu/index.php/lymph/article/view/20450.

Miller, J. (2014). *The roll model*. Las Vegas, NV: Victory Belt Publishing.

Narins, R. S. (2003). *Safe liposuction and fat transfer*. New York, NY: Marcel Dekker.

Nedelec, Bernadette & Lasalle, Léo. (2018). Postburn Itch: A Review of the Literature. Wounds : a compendium of clinical research and practice. 30. E118-E124. Retrieved from: https://www.woundsresearch.com/article/postburn-itch-review-literature

Nolan, P. B., Keeling, S. M., Robitaille, C. A., Buchanan, C. A., & Dalleck, L. C. (2018). The effect of detraining after a period of training on cardiometabolic health in previously sedentary individuals. *International Journal of Environmental Research and Public Health*, 15(10), 2303. doi:10.3390/ijerph15102303. Retrieved from https://www.ncbi.nlm.nih.gov/pmc/articles/PMC6210016.

Ojeh, N., Stojadinovic, O., Pastar, I., Sawaya, A., Yin, N., & Tomic-Canic, M., The effects of caffeine on wound healing, *International Wound Journal*. 2016 Oct;13(5):605–13. doi: 10.1111/iwj.12327. Epub 2014 Jul 8. Retrieved at https://www.ncbi.nlm.nih.gov/pubmed/25041108.

Olaitan, P. B., Chen, I. P., Norris, J. E., Feinn, R., Oluwatosin, O. M., & Reichenberger, E. J. (2011). Inhibitory activities of omega-3 fatty acids and traditional African remedies on keloid fibroblasts. *Wounds: a compendium of clinical research and practice*, 23(4), 97–106. Retrieved from https://www.ncbi.nlm.nih.gov/pmc/articles/PMC3905615.

Olesen, R. M., & Olesen, M. B. (2005). *Cosmetic surgery for dummies*. Hoboken, NJ: Wiley.

Olsen, J. H. H., Oberg, S., & Rosenberg, J. (2019). The effect of compression stocking on leg edema and discomfort during a 3-hour flight: A randomized controlled trial. *European Journal of Internal Medicine*. 2019 Feb 6. pii: S0953-6205(19)30022-6. doi: 10.1016/j.ejim.2019.01.013. Retrieved from https://www.ncbi.nlm.nih.gov/pubmed/30738701.

Oosterveld, F. G. J., Rasker, J. J., Floors, M. et al. (2009). Infrared sauna in patients with rheumatoid arthritis and ankylosing spondylitis. Clinical Rheumatology (2009) 28: 29. https://doi.org/10.1007/s10067-008-0977-y Retrieved from https://link.springer.com/article/10.1007/s10067-008-0977-y

Pazyar N, Yaghoobi R, Kazerouni A, Feily A. Oatmeal in dermatology: A brief review. Indian J Dermatol Venereol Leprol [serial online] 2012. 78:142–5. Available from: http://www.ijdvl.com/text.asp?2012/78/2/142/93629

Perry, A. W. (2007). *Straight talk about cosmetic surgery*. New Haven: Yale University Press.

Plemons, E. (2017). *The look of a woman: Facial feminization surgery and the aims of trans-medicine*. Durham: Duke University Press.

Porcari, J., Ryskey, A., & Foster, C. (2018). The effects of high intensity neuromuscular electrical stimulation on abdominal strength and endurance, core strength, abdominal girth, and perceived body shape and satisfaction. *International Journal of Kinesiology and Sports Science*. 6. 19. 10.7575/aiac.ijkss.v.6n.1p.19. Retrieved from https://journals.aiac.org.au/index.php/IJKSS/article/view/4139/3278.

Kassardjian, N. (n.d.). Post Operative Care. Retrieved from https://www.liposuction.com/post-operative-care-html.

Kraft, K., Kanter, S., & Janik, H. (2013). Safety and effectiveness of vibration massage by deep oscillations: A prospective observational study. *Evidence-based Complementary and Alternative Medicine: eCAM*, 2013, Article ID 679248, 10 pages. doi:10.1155/2013/679248 Retrieved from https://www.ncbi.nlm.nih.gov/pmc/articles/PMC3814103/

Pane, T. (2019). Experience with high-volume buttock fat transfer: A report of 137 cases. *Aesthetic Surgery Journal*, 39(5), 526–532. doi: 10.1093/asj/sjy191. Retrieved from https://academic.oup.com/asj/article/39/5/526/5067487.

Radek K. A., Matthies, A. M., Burns, A. L., Heinrich, S. A., Kovacs, E. J., & DiPietro, L. A. (2005). Acute ethanol exposure impairs angiogenesis and the proliferative phase of wound healing. *American Journal of Physiology-Heart and Circulatory Physiology*. 2005;289:H1084–H1090. Retrieved from https://www.physiology.org/doi/full/10.1152/ajpheart.00080.2005

Rittweger, J. (2010). Vibration as an exercise modality: How it may work, and what its potential might be. *European Journal of Applied Physiology* 108(5), 877–904. doi: 10.1007/s00421-009-1303-3 Retrieved from https://link.springer.com/article/10.1007%2Fs00421-009-1303-3.

Saltz, R. & Ohana, B. Thirteen years of experience with the

endoscopic midface lift, *Aesthetic Surgery Journal*, 32(8), 927–936. doi: 10.1177/1090820X12462714. Retrieved from https://www.ncbi.nlm.nih.gov/pubmed/23110925.

Saint Louis, C. (2010, December 15). Wildly abrasive. *New York Times*. Retrieved from http://www.nytimes.com/2010/12/16/fashion/16Skin.html

Sasada, M., & Guest, P. (2016). *The facelift bible: Including the facelift diaries*. Clinispa Limited.

Schafer, J. (2011). *A patient's guide to liposuction*. Denver, CO: Outskirts Press.

Schaverien, M. V., Munnoch, D. A., & Brorson, H. (2018). Liposuction treatment of lymphedema. *Seminars in Plastic Surgery*, 32(1), 42–47. doi:10.1055/s-0038-1635116. Retrieved from https://www.ncbi.nlm.nih.gov/pmc/articles/PMC5891650.

Schaverien, M. V., Moeller, J. A., & Cleveland, S. D. (2018). Nonoperative treatment of lymphedema. *Seminars in Plastic Surgery*, 32(1), 17–21. doi:10.1055/s-0038-1635119. Retrieved from https://www.ncbi.nlm.nih.gov/pmc/articles/PMC5891656.

Schell, A, Copp, J, Bogie, K.M., & Wetzel, R. Honey-based salve and burdock leaf dressings as an alternative to surgical debridement of a traumatic wound eschar. *Advances in Wound Care*, 8(3), 101–107. doi:10.1089/wound.2018.0806. Retrieved from https://www.ncbi.nlm.nih.gov/pmc/articles/PMC6430982/pdf/wound.2018.0806.pdf.

Shiffman, M. A., & Giuseppe, A. D. (2006). *Liposuction: Principles and practice*. Berlin: Springer-Verlag.

Son, D., & Harijan, A. (2014). Overview of surgical scar prevention and management. *Journal of Korean Medical Science*, 29(6),

751–7. Retrieved from https://www.ncbi.nlm.nih.gov/pmc/articles/PMC4055805.

Sood, A., Granick, M. S., & Tomaselli, N. L. (2014). wound dressings and comparative effectiveness data. *Advances in Wound Care*, 3(8), 511–529. doi:10.1089/wound.2012.0401 Retrieved from https://www.ncbi.nlm.nih.gov/pmc/articles/PMC4121107.

Sotelo-Paz, M. (2016). *Before & After A Guide for Cosmetic Surgery* [Kindle edition]. Retrieved from Amazon.com.

Smith, T. (2017 Jan 27). Are e-cigs safe? Retrieved from https://www.uchealth.org/today/2017/01/27/study-questions-safety-of-e-cigarettes/

Smith, T. J. & Ashar, B. H. (2019). Iron deficiency anemia due to high-dose turmeric. *Cureus*, 11(1), e3858. doi:10.7759/cureus.3858. Retrieved from https://www.ncbi.nlm.nih.gov/pmc/articles/PMC6414192.

Starkey, J. (2015, January 26). The truth about dry brushing and what it does for you. Retrieved from https://health.clevelandclinic.org/2015/01/the-truth-about-dry-brushing-and-what-it-does-for-you.

Stramer, B., Mori, R. & Martin, P. (2007) The inflammation–fibrosis link? A Jekyll and Hyde role for blood cells during wound repair. *Journal of Investigative Dermatology*, 127(5), 1009–1017. Retrieved from https://www.sciencedirect.com/science/article/pii/S0022202X15333534.

The Fitting Room (n.d.) Retrieved from: https://www.designveronique.com/the-fitting-room#section-heading-20

Todd, M., Lay-Flurrie, K., & Drake, J. (2017). Managing ulceration and lymphorrhea in chronic oedema. *British Journal of Community*

Nursing 22(5), S34-S41. doi: 10.12968/bjcn.2017.22.Sup5. S34. Retrieved from http://www.jobstcompressioninstitute.com/uploads/Document-Library/8d4526de3e83a518d1ff7df0f96a42 ec.pdf.

Tummy Tuck. (2018). Retrieved from https://www.smartbeautyguide.com/procedures/body/tummy-tuck.

Tummy Tuck: 8 Tips for a Successful Recovery (2019, Feb. 25). Retrieved from https://www.smartbeautyguide.com/news/body-contouring/tummy-tuck-8-tips-successful-recovery.

Vidal, P., Berner, J. E., & Will, P. A. (2017). Managing complications in abdominoplasty: A literature review. *Archives of Plastic Surgery*, 44(5), 457–468. doi:10.5999/aps.2017.44.5.457. Retrieved from https://www.ncbi.nlm.nih.gov/pmc/articles/PMC5621815.

Ward, A.R. & Shkuratova, N. (2002). Russian electrical stimulation: The early experiments. *Physical therapy* 82(10), 1019–30. Epub 2002/09/28. Retrieved from https://www.ncbi.nlm.nih.gov/pubmed/12350217.

Wear & Care (n.d.) Retrieved from http://www.jobst-usa.com/our-products/wear-care.

White, M. (2017). Application of electric muscle stimulation in acute injuries. Retrieved from https://www.orthoquestpedorthics.com/resources/blog/news/Blog-Entries/2017/01/27/38:application-of-electrical-muscle-stimulation-in-acute-injuries.

White, R. C. (2018). *The stress management workbook: De-stress in 10 minutes or less*. Emeryville, CA: Althea Press.

Wodash A. J. (2013 Sept. 22). Wet-to-dry dressings do not provide moist wound healing. *Journal of the American College of Clinical Wound Specialists* 4(3), 63–66. doi:10.1016/j.jccw.2013.08.001.

Retrieved from https://www.ncbi.nlm.nih.gov/pmc/articles/PMC4511549/pdf/main.pdf.

Wollina, U., Heinig, B., & Nowak, A. (2014). Treatment of elderly patients with advanced lipedema: A combination of laser-assisted liposuction, medial thigh lift, and lower partial abdominoplasty. *Clinical, Cosmetic and Investigational Dermatology* 7, 35–42. doi:10.2147/CCID.S56655. Retrieved from https://www.ncbi.nlm.nih.gov/pmc/articles/PMC3904776.

Wynn, T. A. (2008). Cellular and molecular mechanisms of fibrosis. *Journal of Pathology*, 214(2), 199–210. Retrieved from https://www.ncbi.nlm.nih.gov/pmc/articles/PMC2693329.

Zhao, W., Chen, J., & Chen, W. (2014). Effect of abdominal liposuction on sonographically guided high-intensity focused ultrasound ablation. *Journal of Ultrasound in Medicine* 33(9), 1539–44. Retrieved from https://onlinelibrary.wiley.com/doi/full/10.7863/ultra.33.9.1539.

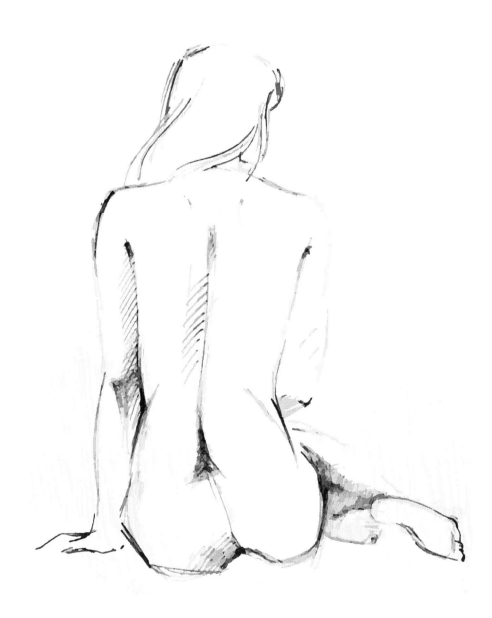

ABOUT THE AUTHOR

Kathleen Lisson is board certified in therapeutic massage and bodywork and is a Certified Lymphedema Therapist. She owns Solace Massage and Mindfulness, has taught classes at IPSB Massage College in San Diego, and is the author of *Lipedema Treatment Guide* and *Swollen, Bloated and Puffy: A Manual Lymphatic Drainage Therapist's Guide to Reducing Swelling in the Face and Body*. Kathleen holds a Bachelors of Applied Science degree in Massage Therapy, and is an NHI (Natural Healing Institute of Naturopathy) Certified Master Aromatherapist, an MMI (McLean Meditation Institute) Certified Meditation Teacher, and an ACE-certified Personal Trainer. She is certified to present Peggy Huddleston's "Prepare for Surgery, Heal Faster" workshop. She was a speaker at the 2018 and 2019 Fat Disorders Resource Society conferences, a keynote speaker at the 2019 MLD UK conference and completed the Lymphedema Therapy Advanced and Review class at the Földi Clinic in Hinterzarten, Germany.

After fourteen years in a high-stress career in public relations for the New York state legislature, Kathleen began her second career as a massage therapist at the nonprofit Adams Avenue Integrative Health, where she partnered with naturopaths, chiropractors, and acupuncturists to provide care to families in the Normal Heights neighborhood in San Diego. She has also volunteered to provide free chair massage to underserved communities in City Heights at Tubman-Chavez Center and the East African Cultural Community Center through the nonprofit Alternative Healing Network.

Kathleen is the author of articles published in *Elephant Journal* and the *Labyrinth Pathways* 10th edition. She has been quoted in the November, 2016 issue of *Prevention magazine*, and online in *Bustle, Consumer Reports, Massage Magazine, Paper, Prevention,* and *Runner's World*.

Social Media:

Http://www.plasticsurgeryrecoveryhandbook.com
Http://www.solacesandiego.com
https://www.facebook.com/
PlasticSurgeryRecoveryHandbook
https://www.instagram.com/
plasticsurgeryrecoveryhandbook/
https://twitter.com/KathleenLisson

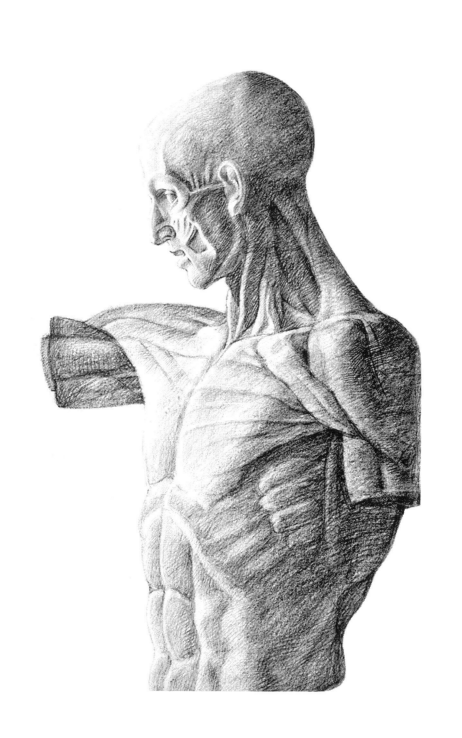

POST-SURGERY DIARY

I recommend you write a few lines about any sign, no matter how small, that you are looking or feeling better today than you were yesterday, a few days ago, or last week. It can even be a nice compliment from a family member or a friend. Looking back on this journal in the future will give you hope that you are recovering well.

Day 1 After Surgery

_____

_____

_____

_____

Day 2 After Surgery

_____

_____

_____

_____

Day 3 After Surgery

_____

_____

_____

_____

Day 4 After Surgery

_____

_____

_____

_____

Day 5 After Surgery

_____

_____

_____

_____

Day 6 After Surgery

_____

_____

_____

_____

Day 7 After Surgery

_____

_____

_____

_____

Day 8 After Surgery

_____

_____

_____

_____

Day 9 After Surgery

_____

_____

_____

Day 10 After Surgery

_____

_____

_____

Day 11 After Surgery

_____

_____

_____

Day 12 After Surgery

_____

_____

_____

_____

Day 13 After Surgery

_____

_____

_____

Day 14 After Surgery

_____

_____

_____

Day 15 After Surgery

_____

_____

_____

Day 16 After Surgery

_____

_____

_____

_____

Day 17 After Surgery

_____

_____

_____

_____

Day 18 After Surgery

_____

_____

_____

_____

Day 19 After Surgery

_____

_____

_____

_____

Day 20 After Surgery

_____

_____

_____

_____

Day 21 After Surgery

_____

_____

_____

_____

Day 22 After Surgery
_____

_____

_____

_____

Day 23 After Surgery
_____

_____

_____

_____

Day 24 After Surgery
_____

_____

_____

_____

Day 25 After Surgery
_____

_____

_____

_____

Day 26 After Surgery

_____

_____

_____

Day 27 After Surgery

_____

_____

_____

Day 28 After Surgery

_____

_____

_____

Day 29 After Surgery

_____

_____

_____

Day 30 After Surgery

_____

_____

_____

_____

Day 31 After Surgery

_____

_____

_____

_____

Day 32 After Surgery

_____

_____

_____

_____

Day 33 After Surgery

_____

_____

_____

_____

Day 34 After Surgery

_____

_____

_____

_____

Day 35 After Surgery

_____

_____

_____

_____

Day 36 After Surgery

_____

_____

_____

_____

Day 37 After Surgery

_____

_____

_____

_____

Day 38 After Surgery

_____

_____

_____

_____

Day 39 After Surgery

_____

_____

_____

Day 40 After Surgery

_____

_____

_____

_____

Printed in Great Britain
by Amazon